THE EVIDENCE-BASED GUIDE TO KIDNEY AND RENAL DIETS

A Guide for Patients, Caregivers and Clinicians

LEE HULL

The Evidence-Based Guide to Kidney and Renal Diets
A Guide for Patients, Caregivers and Clinicians

Published by Kidneyhood.org

First edition, 2024

ISBN 979-8-3411144-9-4

Table of Contents

Foreword

I am a Family Doctor and in 2019 I was pretty healthy but for some reason my kidney function tests became elevated and my cardiologist suggested I see a well-known Nephrologist at a major academic medical center.

When I went to the visit, he surprised me by saying that I had Stage 3 Chronic Kidney Disease (CKD). I asked him how this is treated and he stated that there were not any current treatments nor medications. The basic recommendation was I should eat, sleep and exercise well. I explained that I already do this and he said…..do more. I then asked him the prognosis and he said that in about 3 years I would likely progress to Stage 5 and he could treat with Dialysis and or put me on the kidney transplant list. Not wanting to have 3-5 hour daily sessions hooked up to a dialysis machine nor a kidney transplant, I went home and reread all the journals, websites, and books on CKD I could find.

Since I have been deeply involved in medical innovation for 30 or more years, I started reviewing both the medical and lay literature. To my surprise 3 weeks before, a new 500+ page book called Stopping Kidney Disease was added to Amazon and that began my relationship with Lee Hull who I credit with dramatically changing my life for the better.

Lee has had chronic kidney disease for 25+ years and had never wanted dialysis and had begun reading the world medical literature and traveled extensively to try to figure out a plan to slow or stop kidney disease. I give him tremendous credit for his perseverance, grit and determination for this work. He has probably read and reread more clinical studies than most nephrologists and has used himself as a guinea pig to try different approaches. What is more, he continues this quest not just for himself but for all those in the world who suffer from CKD. He has dedicated his life and even formed a company to provide education and a plan that can improve the way CKD patients are treated.

As new clinical studies and information become available, he clearly wants those with CKD to have the most current medical basis for their treatment of this potentially devastating disease. Therefore, he has written this new book to help both patients and clinicians understand everything about CKD and an approach that can help prevent dialysis and kidney transplants. He has asked me since I am a physician and fellow kidney patient to help edit this book and I gladly accepted. **In my view this book is a MUST READ for CKD patients and clinicians who treat CKD patients.**

In case you are interested in the current status of my kidney disease story, here are the blood study results (which are super according to all physicians who have looked at them). My GFR is still 70% higher than it was five years ago and my BUN and creatinine levels have been normalized.

Kidney Function Tests	Initial Results at Nephrologist 2019	Current 2025 results	Normal values
BUN	33 mg/dL	21 mg/dL	8-27
Creatinine	1.96 mg/dL	1.26 mg/dL	.76-1.27
GFR	33 mL/min/1.73	58 mL/min/1.73	> 59

My progress is due to the Lee Hull developed program that I and over hundreds of CKD patients are currently using in over a dozen countries and that program is detailed in this new great book.

As a physician and as a patient, I would implore you to take the time to get educated on your kidneys and your disease.

Your education is the biggest factor in your future outcome.

—Dr. Jay Rosan

Introduction

This is the first in a series of updates to the Kidneyhood.org book series. After 5 years of working with over 1,000 patients and conducting clinical trials, we have a much better idea of the evidence and information needed by both patients and clinicians to be successful in managing kidney disease.

As always, our goal is to help everyone with chronic kidney disease become healthier and delay or possibly eliminate the need for dialysis or kidney transplant. We want long, active, high-quality lives despite having an incurable disease. Improving our health improves every aspect of our lives.

The main way we can help people improve is through factual education on how your kidneys function, how kidney disease progresses and providing you with the most up to date research and data. **Your education on kidney disease and kidney disease progression is the key that unlocks a better future outcome.**

Mass confusion regarding kidney or renal diets

There is a kind of *mass confusion* about dietary management of kidney[1] disease. We will discuss the reasons for this confusion, but I see no reason to allow this confusion to persist as it is so damaging to patients. Data on different kidney diets and related studies have been published for decades. Collectively, hundreds of studies on over a million patients give us very good evidence about what we can expect with different approaches to kidney disease management. I hope we can end most of the confusion by putting verified, validated and vetted information in one convenient book.

This *mass confusion* is caused by several factors.

Understanding how this craziness got started and why it has been allowed to prosper and grow will make you a better and more careful consumer of this kind of information.

First, diets, dietary advice(paid or unpaid), diet books, websites, and so on have no regulations or requirements to be effective, safe, accurate, tested, proven, provide complete nutrition or anything at all. Dietary advice is not regulated in any way. Patients falsely assume that because something is published, printed, paid for, or on the web, it must have some evidence behind it. Nothing could be further from the truth. To illustrate this point, over 30 kidney/renal diet books are listed on Amazon.

---

1   We are using the kidney in this book, but *renal* means exactly the same thing.

com, only 2 have any human data behind them, and 1 of those 2 has been clinically proven. Using this example, 97% of dietary advice has never been tested or evaluated in actual kidney patients.

A second contributing cause is that no accepted or common standards exist on how to evaluate effectiveness of different dietary or nutritional approaches to kidney disease. Drugs have a tough approval process that is the same for all drugs. Diet-related issues have no standards. It's almost impossible to determine if something is effective when no one knows how to measure effectiveness and testing is not required. When 90% of drugs fail to get approval from the FDA because they don't meet rigid standards, you can bet 90%+ of dietary approaches would fail as well using the same standards.

A third factor is that online misinformation and misleading marketing is growing at an exponential rate compared to factual, verifiable information. A mini-industry exists selling unproven products, dietary services and content to desperate kidney patients. Each year they get better and better with claims and marketing. A big part of your education is that you are the only form of quality control in this unregulated area.

A fourth factor is that recommendations or guidance from reputable kidney-related organizations and clinicians can be conflicting or vague, further adding to our confusion. What happens when the experts don't agree? We will cover these in the book and what the recommendations are in each relevant chapter.

A fifth factor is our doctors/nephrologists will normally say kidney diets are not effective despite online claims to the contrary. Very few if any dietary approaches have proven to produce good outcomes and your doctor knows this fact. If a patient sees three different dietitians/nutritionists they will get three different recommendations and none of those recommendations will have been tested in humans. It's no one's fault to be clear, but it's an incredibly frustrating experience for patients.

Last, kidney disease is a complicated, systemic and often counterintuitive disease that science still does not completely understand. One issue this book documents very well is that we are still in the infancy of dietary management of kidney disease despite 50 years of published research. We will show you how to deal with this issue later in the book.

The two cures for this confusion are education and objective standards.

The heavy lift: your education

It's a very heavy lift to educate patients to a point in which they can successfully manage kidney disease, but it can be done. We see this every day at work. It does take time, effort and motivation on our part. However, it's also very clear that patients who don't take the time to get educated have poor, if not impossible odds of managing kidney disease successfully. We see this daily as well. Medical doctors with kidney disease are the most successful group of kidney patients in our program due to education on kidneys and kidney disease progression.

An objective cure for this confusion

The cure for the dietary confusion is education and applying the same objective standards to all kidney diets. Objective standards should reflect our goals as kidney patients trying to beat or slow down a currently incurable disease. **Put another way, if we want to know if a particular diet helps our kidney disease, we need to measure all diets the same way.**

We will show you down-to-the-milligram evidence available in 2024 on different approaches to kidney disease management. Diets, nutrition, changes in lifestyle and patient education are not drugs, to be sure, but a rigid and objective standard like the kind drugs follow would eliminate almost all of the confusion regarding kidney disease diets overnight, as you will see.

An evidence-based guide in three parts

In the first part of this book, we will educate you on types of scientific studies, blood tests and terms you should understand, and a brief overview of kidney disease. We need to cover some basics first, so the next parts make sense and are easier to read and understand. We will also decide how to judge the information we find in Parts 2 and 3. (This part is for patients more than clinicians.)

The second part of this book is based on large-scale reviews and studies on established groups of kidney diets. Most of this information is considered to be proven fact due to the amount of data and consistency of conclusions. After reading the second section of the book, you will know more about kidney diets than anyone you have ever met. You need this education to better understand dietary options and what real studies suggest is possible or impossible.

The last section of the book is sharing what we have learned in the first 5 years of Kidneyhood.org, working to finally achieve a clinically proven program to manage kidney disease. Hopefully, we are in the early stages of documenting the **first real breakthrough in kidney diets and kidney disease management in decades**. After 25+ years as a kidney patient myself and now working with thousands of patients, we have a clear understanding of who improves and why they improve. We also have a good understanding of how kidney disease progresses and what it takes to properly deal with the drivers of kidney disease progression. Much of the last part falls into emerging evidence and theory, so I wanted to keep it separate. As a result, you'll find established facts in the first two-thirds and new evidence and new technology in the last third of the book.

The big goal is a better future for all of us

If we all had the same education on kidney disease and current evidence, I believe we could save millions of lives over time, greatly reduce the number of patients on dialysis or waiting on a transplant, and extend the useful life of most patients' kidneys for many years—even decades. We would live in a world where getting great healthcare and extending the useful life of our kidneys is an everyday thing. Confusion would be rare instead of an everyday thing. I personally believe we are in the early stages of a revolution in kidney disease management based on our study results and feedback from hundreds of patients. To get involved, get yourself as educated as possible on the evidence for kidney diets and clear understanding of how kidney disease progresses.

Thank you

I want to thank everyone who participated in our studies and the physicians, clinical coordinators and statisticians who help us collect, evaluate, and write past and currently ongoing pilot studies. We are attempting multiple studies each year now to add to our body of information as rapidly as possible. I also want to thank the researchers and physicians who published research on dietary management of kidney disease. All studies have great value and expand our knowledge base.

My sincere hope is that you, your caregivers, and medical professionals will learn enough in this book that you change your entire future as it relates to your health and kidney disease.

Please reach out to us at support@kidneyhood.org or visit our website (www.kidney-hood.org) if we can help in any way.

One reminder: You should always be under the care of a qualified physician.

Chapter 1

How to Read and Understand Medical Studies So We Have a Better Chance of Extending the Useful Life of Our Kidneys

In an effort to bring us up to date on facts and away from outdated data, I wanted to use the first chapter to explain the studies and metastudies used later in the book. Understanding how scientists and researchers approach studies and trials will help us understand which facts to trust.

How do we, as patients, obtain accurate, factual, verified information that is relevant to us?

We see this as one of our roles. We need to provide you with the best, most up-to-date information in an easy-to-read guide. We need to put the data in your hands and educate you on the evidence. We are trying to write one guide for both patients and clinicians to use as a reference.

It's a bit tedious in some chapters as small details really matter, but I will try to keep it as simple as possible. A little extra effort put into understanding your kidneys and disease can yield life-changing outcomes. Please read or reread every chapter as needed. You can also reach out to us at support@kidneyhood.org with any questions.

Let's dive into separating fact from fiction.

Let's start with what a *metastudy, meta-analysis,* or *systematic review* is as a form of evidence.

Metastudies, meta-analyses, and systematic reviews are all similar, so we treat these as one concept here. These large studies normally consider all available individual studies on a selected topic.

For example, if we assume 80 relevant studies exist on a specific topic, then all 80 studies will be considered for the metastudy. Studies that appear to have a bias or are considered low quality are normally excluded from the metastudy analysis. What we are left with is an analysis of the highest quality studies with the least amount of bias.

Let's assume only 35 studies (out of 80 studies) met the criteria for being high quality and lacking bias. Only these studies will be used to draw conclusions. Anyone can read the metastudy and find out what the best 35 studies (again, in this example) found as a large group of high-quality studies.

In addition, published studies and articles (including metastudies) also go through a peer-review process where other scientists or physicians review and evaluate the studies before publication. The reputations of the authors and the reviewers depend on publishing good science—if they don't have good reputations, they can't get funding from the government or universities to do more research.

To provide you with the best and most current evidence, we will use metastudies like meta-analyses and systematic reviews when possible. Individual studies will be used when larger studies are unavailable. We use the latest research available. Many studies are from the last 5 years, so this will be new data that patients and clinicians have never seen before.

Using metastudies and reviews allows us to use a few larger studies that normally cover decades of individual studies to form an opinion based on the strength of the evidence or findings.

A secondary factor—but maybe even more important—is when multiple metastudies or systematic reviews exist on a single issue and all of the studies agree or come to a similar conclusion. Then this is some of the best evidence we can use to form our own opinion. Assume 3–5 large-scale metastudies on a topic are all in agreement with no conflicting opinions. This represents incredibly high-quality evidence for us to base health care decisions on. However, sometimes studies may conflict with each other, and that's a red flag for us to dig deeper or be more careful in our research.

Another major reason for using these large studies and reviews is to help combat misinformation (especially online), misleading marketing, out of data information and ignorance about nutritional approaches to kidney disease. Anyone can dismiss a single study, but multiple metastudies and reviews covering thousands of patients are hard to argue against. To help deal with this problem, I put dozens of vetted, verified, and peer-reviewed research articles hidden away in niche medical journals into your hands. My goal is to live in a world where care is much better for all, and that starts with your education.

Chapter 2

Kidney Disease 101

Section 1: Kidney Words or Terms and Theories to Be Aware of Going Forward

Most of us see the terms in this chapter on our blood tests but may not be sure what these tests mean or what the tests are telling us about our current health or our predicted outcomes for the future.

There are a few things you should be aware of when you think of kidney-related tests or those related to kidney diets.

Everything is a measure of waste products.

The first lesson I want to share is that everything in the kidney world is largely a measure of waste products or waste byproducts because healthy kidneys remove waste well, but unhealthy kidneys don't. Waste byproducts are the excesses that remain after dietary consumption and must be removed by our kidneys(in most cases). These waste byproducts can be very toxic to us if levels get high enough.

Our kidney-related lab tests are all based on the amounts of waste products in our bloodstream. There are no exceptions to this rule. Keep this in mind while you are reading this book.

Estimated glomerular filtration rate (eGFR) or glomerular filtration rate (GFR): These are very similar measures of your kidney's ability to filter waste products from your bloodstream. As higher amounts of wastes build up in your bloodstream, your GFR will go down indicating a lowered ability to properly filter and excrete waste products. The possible GFR range is 0–120 (hypothetically). We are considered to have kidney disease when GFR drops below 60. GFR or eGFR can be calculated in different ways using different blood tests, but all GFRs are measures of waste products in our bloodstream.

Creatinine: This is a waste byproduct primarily from muscle breakdown and, to a lesser extent, from food intake. Muscle breakdown occurs every day as our bodies repair, recycle, or build muscle tissue. As creatinine levels rise, it is a sign that our kidneys are not able to remove waste byproducts faster than our bodies create them. Creatinine levels may also increase if you start exercising heavily as more muscle tissue is broken down. The normal ranges for creatinine are 0.7–1.3 mg/dL (61.9–114.9 µmol/L) for men and 0.6–1.1 mg/dL (53–97.2 µmol/L) for women.

Blood urea nitrogen (BUN) is a direct measurement of dietary protein intake vs your kidney's ability to filter waste products produced by dietary protein intake. Dietary protein means the protein in the foods/drinks you consume. All forms of dietary protein (plant- and animal-based) contain nitrogen which is the waste byproduct from consuming protein. Our bodies must remove the nitrogen waste component before many amino acids can be used by our body to build muscles and do other important jobs. These nitrogen-based waste products are toxic in high levels and cause both kidney and heart disease to progress at a faster rate. BUN levels are also predictive of our future outcomes. Normal BUN levels are 6–24 mg/dL (2.1–8.5 mmol/L), but ideal BUN levels are well below 20 mg/dL.

If your BUN levels are above the normal ranges or rising, you are eating more dietary and/or supplemental protein than your kidneys can handle.

Cystatin C: A newer test—**cystatin C**—is a measure of waste products from cells. Healthy kidneys remove these wastes and keep levels normal. However, diseased kidneys may not be able to keep up, and cystatin C starts to build up, which lowers your calculated GFR (when cystatin C is used to calculate GFR). A normal cystatin C level is between 0.53–0.95 mg/L, but this can vary depending on the laboratory method used. The normal range should be printed in your blood tests. For adults over 50, the normal range is a little higher , 0.58–1.02 mg/L.

Together, different waste products or different waste product tests give a measurement of kidney disease progression and the severity of our disease. If levels of these waste products become too high, dialysis is used to reduce the amount of these toxic waste products. Dialysis is a procedure to remove waste products from the blood when the kidneys stop working properly. It often involves diverting blood to a machine to be cleaned daily or at least 3 times per week.

A protein source with reduced waste products

The next term is not used for blood tests, but it is a term you need to be familiar with going forward. ***Keto acid analogs*** are used in very low protein diets (VLPD) as a protein supplement to provide protein nutrition with reduced waste products.

Keto acid analogs, also called keto analogs or keto acids, are often abbreviated as KA.[2] Keto acid analogs are essential amino acids with the toxic nitrogen waste component removed. Essential amino acids are the ones our body cannot make and must be provided by dietary intake.

Keto acid analogs offer a method of getting protein nutrition without the nitrogen waste workload as the waste component (nitrogen) is removed in a lab, so your body doesn't have to remove it. In fact, the entire reason keto acid analogs were developed is to reduce the nitrogen levels we see as blood urea nitrogen or BUN on our blood tests and reduce the workload on the kidney. The higher the nitrogen content of keto acid analogs, the more you are contributing to waste byproducts that show up in blood tests as blood urea nitrogen.

However, the potential benefits of keto acid analogs may extend well beyond protein nutrition according to new studies, so the distinction between authentic or real keto acid analogs compared to other forms of protein supplementation is very important. There will be more on this in Chapter 8.

Section 2: Reputable Global Kidney Disease Guidance: Sources to Be Aware Of

I also want you to be aware of reputable sources. Both reports listed below are very good sources of information on managing kidney disease and contain recommendations that we consider best practices.

Kidney Disease Outcome Quality Initiative or KDOQI: This joint report is published by the National Kidney Foundation and the American Academy of Nutrition and Dietetics in the American Journal of Kidney Diseases.[1] The KDOQI is a lengthy document (100+ pages with 500+ citations), so only the most important parts will be mentioned. Much of the KDOQI deals with dialysis patients, which are not covered in this book. The KDOQI is the closest thing we have to a form of quality control for dietary management of kidney disease.

You can download or view the entire KDOQI here:

2020 Kidney Disease Outcome Quality Initiatives (KDOQI) update

https://doi.org/10.1053/j.ajkd.2020.05.006

---

2   Keto acid analogs have nothing to do with keto or ketosis-related diets.

Kidney Disease Improving Global Outcomes (KDIGO) is another excellent resource.[2] KDIGO published guidelines are similar to the KDOQI above. KDIGO is a non-profit organization made up of clinicians from around the world. Only relevant parts of the KDIGO will be mentioned. The KDIGO is updated every few years just like the KDOQI, and the most recent update was in 2024.

You can download or view it here:

https://kdigo.org/wp-content/uploads/2024/03/KDIGO-2024-CKD-Guideline.pdf

Both the KDIGO and the KDOQI are excellent resources, but the recommendations can be conflicting and somewhat vague when it comes to dietary issues. Unfortunately, this adds to both patient and clinician confusion. Education and objective standards are going to help us sort through conflicting recommendations.

Should a standard for effectiveness exist for kidney diets?

The expectation we follow in this book is that we, as patients and clinicians, would always want the most proven, up-to-date and safe options to help us slow kidney disease progression and improve our overall health.

An objective standard is the missing link we need to guide patients and clinicians.

An objective standard would allow us to separate the effective from the ineffective and spend our time, money, and effort on the best dietary approach for our situation by measuring the things that actually matter to us patients. An objective standard would allow clinicians and organizations to clearly agree or disagree on what works and what doesn't. Objective standards or regulations exist for almost every form of healthcare except dietary recommendations.

The lack of an objective standard is the single biggest contributor to dietary confusion and misinformation for both patients and clinicians.

I am going to repeat this for emphasis:

The lack of an objective standard is the single biggest contributor to dietary confusion and misinformation for both patients and clinicians.

As you will see in this book, applying 2 simple but important standards eliminates almost all confusion regarding kidney and renal diets. We go from very confusing to almost no confusion when standards are applied.

I will try to point out some red flags for patients and clinicians as we go. These red flags are issues you should pay special attention to if you run into them. We as patients (myself included) often overlook every red flag or potential problem because we want something to work. We are so desperate for any kind of improvement; we can't see the obvious in many cases. Many of the things I tried were doomed from the start and could never have worked. However, I didn't understand that at the time, and I didn't know how to look at the research in those days.

No guard rails

Your doctor is a guardrail when it comes to prescription drugs. Your doctor stands between you and prescription drugs. If drugs are not effective or have too many side effects, your doctor will stop use of these drugs. You also cannot access prescription drugs without a doctor's prescription.

There are no guard rails when it comes to diets, supplements, foods, alternative medicine, online information, etc. You are the only guard rail in unregulated areas. You can do whatever you want in this unregulated area. In many cases, patients are using diets and taking supplements that have the potential to accelerate kidney or heart disease progression. Remember, no one is going to tap you on the shoulder and say "You know, what you are doing could never work or may harm you." Education and standards are the guardrails to keep you on the road to improving.

Diets can be as effective, if not more effective, than drugs

Limiting salt to 1,500 mg per is just as effective as blood pressure medications. New studies show that even if you wait until age 60 to start a better diet, you can still add 8–9 years to your life. If you are 80, you may still add 3.5 years to your life. Imagine if a prescription drug added 8–9 years to your life; it would be the greatest breakthrough in medical history. Everyone would be taking this drug, but that drug already exists, and it's improving your diet and lifestyle. These studies were on normal populations, not kidney patients. However, it is likely that kidney patients get even more benefits from successful diets than normal populations. The reason is we have more problems to solve and more accelerated disease rates.

As part of your education, you should understand that diets or dietary improvements may be more effective than prescription drugs in many cases. Many issues common to kidney patients have no available drug treatments to help us, so dietary intake is our only form of control in many cases. The idea that what you eat or drink on a daily basis doesn't matter or doesn't change your future is wrong, dead wrong as you will see.

Effective diets are here today, you don't have to wait for a future breakthrough to add years to your life. This is true whether you are a kidney patient or not.

Chapter 3

Primary Goals of Kidney Diets

Let's start by focusing on the only possible goal for kidney diets.

Your kidneys cannot heal or regrow like other organs. Once parts of your kidneys are damaged, those parts of your kidney never function properly again.[3] Claims to restore, rejuvenate, reverse, cure, or regrow kidneys are largely fraudulent, scam-type claims. We only see these kinds of claims on the internet or on products that are not regulated, but we never see them in medical journals or from reputable organizations. **These kinds of claims are clearly red flags, as they are impossible with current medical science.** Because we cannot regrow or heal our kidneys, the primary purpose of kidney diets can only be to slow the loss of our remaining kidney function.

It makes things a lot simpler when we know exactly what our goal is.

Our real goal is to slow kidney disease progression to a rate slower than normal kidney disease progression. We can't completely stop or cure kidney disease today, so the only realistic option is to try to slow disease progression. Our goal is progression so slow that disease progression is almost not measurable.

For this reason, we are going to focus on the rates of kidney disease progression and how different dietary approaches may speed up or slow down rates of kidney disease progression.

Let's start with a quick review of how kidneys function.

Brief overview of kidney functions

I want to make sure everyone has the same basic information about kidney functions before we go forward. Let's see how these functions appear in kidney patients.

1. **Waste removal:** As discussed, your kidneys remove waste products from your bloodstream so they can be excreted in urine. When your kidney function starts to fail, your ability to remove these toxic waste products starts to decrease. These waste products show up on your blood tests as creatinine, blood urea nitrogen (BUN), cystatin C and GFR.

2. **Fluid balance:** Kidneys maintain the correct fluid balance by excreting or retaining liquids as needed. Swelling will become more common as your kidney function declines over time. High sodium and low albumin (a protein made by the liver) are 2 common causes of swelling in kidney patients.

3. **Vitamins and minerals:** Kidneys also regulate the balance of vitamins and minerals like sodium, potassium, hydrogen, calcium, phosphorus, magnesium, and bicarbonate. As our kidney function decreases, it gets harder to keep things in balance. Certain vitamins can build up or become deficient. Vitamins and mineral nutrition for us is kind of like a Goldilocks situation—we need to have each vitamin and mineral just right to make up for our kidneys' reduced ability to keep vitamins and minerals in the normal ranges.

4. **Blood pressure control:** Your kidneys produce the hormones that help maintain blood pressure. As your kidney function decreases, so does your ability to maintain good blood pressure control. Prescription blood pressure medications for hypertensive kidney patients are considered a best practice.[2] High blood pressure damages the smallest parts of our kidney's filtering system.

5. **Red blood cell production** is controlled by a hormone made by your kidneys. Hormone production drops with kidney function decline. Many patients get anemia as a result. A hormone shot is given to many kidney patients to stimulate red blood cell production. Red blood cells bring oxygen to every part of the body.

6. **Healthy bones:** Kidneys maintain healthy bones by controlling vitamin D, calcium, and magnesium levels. Vitamin D is commonly supplemented in kidney patients, but care must be used as too much vitamin D can be harmful. Too little Vitamin D is also harmful.

7. **Making urine:** Your kidneys selectively reabsorb 99% of all fluids they process back into the blood, and the remaining 1% is excreted in the form of urine. We normally think of excretion or urine with kidneys, but 99% of fluids are reabsorbed to keep our bodies in the optimal range for hydration, vitamin and mineral levels. As our disease progresses and our GFR/eGFR declines, it gets harder and harder for our kidneys to maintain normal levels of everything. We don't excrete some things fast enough, and we don't retain enough of other things to maintain normal levels.

Your kidneys keep everything in normal ranges and maintain homeostasis for your entire body. Your kidneys are connected to every part of your body.

Your kidneys are the most vascular organ in your body, besides your heart. Heart health and kidney health go hand in hand. Heart disease is the number one killer of kidney patients.[4] Specifically, vascular calcification is the leading cause of death for kidney disease patients.[5,6] Kidney disease is considered a perfect storm for accelerating heart disease, so taking care of our kidneys will help our hearts and improve our chances of living a long life.

Most accurate question: How far can I get on 200,000 nephrons?
Your kidneys contain tiny structures that clean your blood. They're called nephrons, and each one has 2 main parts: a filter (the glomerulus) and a small reabsorption tube (the tubule). For this example, we will assume you start with 1 million nephrons with normal, healthy kidneys. Let's assume your GFR is 30 today. That represents 300,000 working nephrons in this hypothetical example. We started with at least 1 million working nephrons when our kidneys were healthy, but we have lost 70% of our kidney function.

Let's further assume most patients will start dialysis when their GFR is below 10 with just 100,000 working nephrons.

The difference between today (300,000 working nephrons, GFR of 30) and dialysis (100,000 working nephrons, GFR of 10) is 200,000 working nephrons. Each year, we lose more nephrons that will not grow back or heal. **The entire point of kidney diets is to preserve or slow the loss of the remaining 200,000 nephrons for as long as possible.**

We need real evidence that any kidney diets, books, supplements, dietary consultants, etc. help us make our remaining nephrons last as long as possible.

How we damage nephrons

Kidney disease usually looks like slow damage to our kidneys that occurs over many years. This damage is often called sclerosis or fibrosis, which basically means our microscopic filters and tubules are being scarred over time. Our kidneys can be scarred by something floating around in our bloodstream in high levels like blood urea nitrogen (BUN) or by some other part of our body that is not working correctly (like high blood pressure). As our microscopic nephron filters are scarred over time, this leads to a reduced ability to filter and excrete waste products, like nitrogen, which show up on our blood tests as blood urea nitrogen or BUN. Frothy or bubbly urine is a sign of protein in the urine. This happens because our tiny, scarred filters are letting protein leak through when protein should have been retained in the body's blood. Our ability to reabsorb what is needed gets slowly worse each year as kidney disease progresses, as does the ability to produce certain hormones.

As our health gets slightly worse each year, nephron loss speeds up due to more complications and more extremes in our blood and urine tests. A kind of snowball effect happens that takes greater and greater forces, or changes in our health, to counteract as the disease progresses.

In summary, kidney disease is slow damage or scarring that occurs over time. Once the damage occurs, it cannot be healed. This is an important fact as managing a disease in which damage is ongoing and permanent begs for the earliest possible intervention. <u>In fact, if any disease warrants the earliest possible intervention, it's kidney disease because our kidneys cannot regrow. Once function is lost, it's normally lost forever.</u>

By allowing ourselves to get sicker and allowing our test results to worsen over time, we are feeding the fires of kidney disease progression. What begins as a small spark from a small issue can quickly escalate to a fire that can take 20 years off our life.

Genetic kidney disease diseases (like polycystic kidney disease and a few others) are different, but this will apply to most of us. Some forms of kidney diseases are autoimmune and can go into remission. The same best practices for traditional kidney patients also appear to improve outcomes for autoimmune forms of kidney disease.

How do we preserve nephrons or slow kidney disease progression?

We will give you a master class on this subject in the last third of the book, but basically, the way we improve our health and hopefully slow kidney disease progression is by effectively treating or managing all of the drivers of kidney disease. We are going to take our foot off the gas and apply the brakes by taking time to get healthier. For example, if our blood pressure is uncontrolled and higher than normal, kidney disease progresses faster. However, if blood pressure is under control, then the speed of kidney disease progression should slow as well. There are literally dozens of factors contributing to how fast your disease progresses, and we have to effectively manage each one. This topic is covered in depth in the last third of the book.

Kidney disease causes very specific nutritional problems, but many of these problems can be solved by an integrated and coordinated dietary approach. We will look at the evidence on how well different approaches manage these nutritional problems in Part 2.

Now that we understand the slow decline that is kidney disease, let's find a way to quantify or measure these issues to set a basic standard for kidney diets.

Chapter 4

Measuring Kidney Diets by Predicted Outcomes—What Will Happen to Us in the Future?

We need a way to measure the effectiveness of kidney diets based on how they change what happens to us in the future (like will we need dialysis sooner or later if we eat a certain way). The scientific way to say it is a standard measure of effectiveness to evaluate diets using information that has been proven predictive of future outcomes.

We want to focus on the issues that give us the best futures, but we also need to use indicators or tests that every patient has access to and can understand without a medical degree.

<u>If the only possible goal for kidney diets is to slow disease progression, then that is exactly how we should evaluate kidney diets.</u>

Trajectory of your GFR as a predictive tool

Let's start with the trajectory of your GFR or how it changes over time—whether it gets better or worse. Almost all blood tests will include GFR or eGFR, so you can see the changes in your GFR over time easily. Most of us can see this data and graph the trajectory online though through an online patient portal. Pay special attention to how steep the line is—this tells us how much GFR is falling between tests. If you don't have this set up, ask your doctor's office to help you make an online account that will help you track your test results over time.

The amount of annual loss (the trend) of kidney function matters much more than your current GFR when predicting your future with kidney disease. This is a very important concept.

The easy way to think about this is that the faster your GFR is dropping each year, the sicker you are getting each year, and the faster you are losing remaining nephrons. <u>The trajectory of your GFR is almost 2 times more important than your actual GFR in predicting your future outcome.</u>

First study on how important GFR trending is in kidney disease

CKD progression prediction in a diverse US population: A machine-learning model (2023)[7]

Aoki J, Kaya C, Khalid O, et al (9 authors)

Number of Patients: 110,264 over 5 years. Initial eGFR between 15–89 mL/min/1.73 m^2

Conclusion: "Using machine-learning techniques on a diverse US population, this cohort study aimed to address this deficiency [that there is no good way to predict how fast kidneys will fail] and found that a 5-year risk prediction model for CKD progression was accurate. The most important predictor of progressive decline in kidney function was the eGFR slope, followed by the urine albumin-creatinine ratio and serum albumin slope."

Easy-to-Read Summary: This study found that GFR slope or trajectory is roughly twice as effective as our current GFR in predicting future outcomes with kidney disease using an AI model.

Second study linking worsening kidney blood studies to worse outcomes

Estimated glomerular filtration rate, albuminuria, and adverse outcomes: An individual-participant data meta-analysis (2023)[8]

Grams ME, Coresh J, Matsushita K, et al (80 authors)

Number of Patients: 27,503,140 with eGFR based on creatinine, 720,736 with eGFR based on creatinine and cystatin C, and 9,067,753 with albuminuria from 1980 to 2021

Conclusions: "Lower eGFR based on creatinine alone, lower eGFR based on creatinine and cystatin C, and more severe UACR [urine albumin-creatinine ratio] were each associated with increased rates of 10 adverse outcomes, including adverse kidney outcomes, cardiovascular diseases, and hospitalizations."

Easy-to-Read Summary: eGFR can be measured several ways, but this very large meta-analysis (with many patients) shows that no matter which measurement method is used, worsening eGFR, cystatin C and urine albumin-creatinine ratio (uACR) are all associated with worse outcomes. No matter which measure was used, trajectory matters.

Data from over 30 million patients was used in this study, so it's trustworthy. I wanted to mention this as some patients get hung up on the type of blood test used, but it really does not matter. The trajectory of these tests (how much they change over time) is what matters, not which test was used.

Third study that shows trending in GFR is important

Evaluating glomerular filtration rate slope as a surrogate end point for ESKD in clinical trials: An individual participant meta-analysis of observational data (2019)[9]

Grams ME, Sang Y, Ballew SH, et al (21 authors)

Number of patients: 3,758,551 with baseline eGFR $\geq$ 60 mL/min/1.73 m^2 and 122,664 participants with eGFR < 60 mL/min/1.73 m^2 followed for an average of 4.2 years

Results: "Slower eGFR decline by 0.75 mL/min per year over 2 years was associated with lower risk of ESRD [end-stage renal disease] in participants with baseline eGFR $\geq$60 and eGFR <60 mL/min."

Conclusions: "Slower decline in eGFR was associated with lower risk of subsequent ESRD, even in participants with eGFR $\geq$60, but those with the highest risk would be expected to benefit the most."

Easy-to-Read Summary: Slowing disease trajectory or progression by less than 1 GFR point per year (0.75 GFR points) was associated with lower future risks of kidney failure. This was true for patients with GFR above or below 60. Changing the trend or trajectory (even a little) can improve future outcomes.

This is one of many studies documenting the benefits of early intervention in stage 3 kidney disease. There were 3+ million patients in this meta-analysis.

Fourth study that once again validated the importance of GFR trend

Trajectory of estimated glomerular filtration rate and malnourishment predict mortality and kidney failure in older adults with chronic kidney disease (2021)[10]

Weng SC, Chen CM, Chen YC, Wu MJ, Tarng DC (5 authors)

Number of Patients: 3,948 patients

Methods: "The trajectory of eGFR is a potential surrogate marker to demonstrate the causal relationship among muscle mass, aging changes in the kidneys, renal survival, and patient mortality."

Discussion: "In conclusion, eGFR trajectories were shown to be a valuable prognostic indicator for predicting outcomes in older adults with CKD. An integrated kidney disease care program could have a notable beneficial effect on patients' mortality and kidney failure, based on a comparison with gradual eGFR decline. <u>Increasing eGFR trajectory in the later period was shown to be a high-risk factor for kidney failure in older CKD patients.</u> These phenomena may be due to multimorbidity, abnormal BMI status, and malnutrition."

Easy- to-Read Summary: This individual study shows the relationship between GFR trajectory and other health concerns like weight (BMI), malnutrition, multiple health issues (multimorbidity), muscle mass, and death (mortality rates). Your GFR trajectory is related to all these health issues. You will see this theme later in the book.

This study also documents the benefits of slowing disease progression as measured by GFR trajectories and the relationship to overall health.

<u>The trajectory, slope, or annual change of your GFR is a proxy for how fast you are losing nephrons. Keep this in mind when you are reading the chapters on different dietary approaches to kidney disease.</u>

GFR trajectories and future outcome

If the only real goal of kidney diets is to slow the loss of our remaining kidney function, we can look at the GFR trajectory results of different kidney diets. This should be a very accurate indicator of the future benefit of these diets.

<u>*Did I change the trajectory of my GFR enough to change my future outcome?* This is the right question.</u>

We are looking for a clinically or statistically significant change in the trajectory of our GFR, not minor improvements. As patients, we often do things like *give up red meat* or *go vegetarian* in an attempt to extend the useful life of our kidneys without understanding these kinds of changes have no documented or proven history of improving our outcomes. Using GFR trajectory as an objective measure clears up any confusion almost immediately.

What we like about this measure is that we get a simple tool to cut through bad, outdated and misleading information with a single indicator (GFR slope or annual loss) that every patient and clinician has access to. Ideally, we would want any diet to slow kidney disease to a rate slower than normal disease progression rates. Can a certain diet slow kidney disease progression to rates slower than normal rates of disease progression? To know, we need to first define what is normal and what's not normal.

Age-related loss versus active disease progression

A 1-year GFR loss of more than -3% is widely considered to be active kidney disease progression. Less than -3% loss may be normal age-related loss of kidney function and may not meet the criteria for active disease progression.[2]

Some variations in GFR or eGFR test results are normal, but the trajectory over time is what matters. Your doctor will help you determine if loss in GFR is age-related or related to active kidney disease progression using multiple test results.

In the big picture, the higher the GFR loss rate, the worse the future outcome will be. While active kidney disease can be described as a >-3% drop in GFR or eGFR, we also need to know when outcomes really start to get bad. Annual declines in GFR >-7.5% lead to the worst outcomes or the bottom 25% of expected outcomes. This is the group we want to avoid being in at all costs.[11]

For this book, we will assume any dietary approaches that cause patient results to fall within the range of -3% and -7.5% annual GFR loss are not having the desired effect of slower kidney disease progression. Kidney disease is still progressing at a rate within the normal disease progression rates.

Any 1-year GFR loss between 0% and -3% is very good. Kidney disease progression is slow enough that the person may no longer meet the criteria for active kidney disease progression. This group would have a better-than-average future outcome. We would consider this to be a successful approach to kidney disease management. **In many ways, this should be the minimum standard for kidney diets to meet in terms of proving effectiveness.**

An increase in GFR or eGFR is so rare that we could not find any related studies on outcomes. For example, GFR or eGFR going from 30 to 40 has not been studied in the past, as these kinds of gains or improvements did not exist in the past. We are tracking outcomes right now to add to this data. Being in this group should put us in the best future outcome, but keep in mind this is new and early data. A flat or increase in GFR should put us in the best group for future outcomes, but this is only true if the gains in GFR can be maintained for years to come.

Blood urea nitrogen (BUN) and future outcomes

BUN is easier to evaluate than GFR, as BUN has normal ranges printed on every blood test. GFR does not have a normal range. The ability of a kidney diet to return BUN level to within the normal range is what matters to us. **Normal is where we get the best future outcomes**.

The normal range for BUN is 6–24 mg/dL (2.1–8.5 mmol/L).

High BUN levels are a strong predictor of many bad things to come. If we break patients into quartiles (groups), the patients in the quartile with the lowest BUN levels have a much better future outcome with kidney disease. Protein-related waste products like BUN are highly toxic to us and will kill us if these levels get high enough. The primary or original purpose of dialysis was to lower levels of these nitrogenous waste products which was—and is— lifesaving.

First study that shows the importance of BUN for kidney health

Blood urea nitrogen is independently associated with renal outcomes in Japanese patients with stage 3–5 chronic kidney disease: A prospective observational study (2019)[12]

Seki M, Nakayama M, Sakoh T, et al (10 authors)

Number of patients: 459 patients with CKD stage 3–5

Conclusions: "Higher BUN levels were associated with adverse renal outcomes independent of the eGFR, suggesting that BUN may be a useful marker for predicting kidney disease progression."

Note on this study: The quartile with the highest BUN levels were almost 100% on dialysis at the end of the 100-month study; in contrast, over 70% of patients in the group with the lowest BUN levels avoided dialysis over this time period, a little over 8 years.

Easy-to-Read Summary: Higher BUN levels meant that people were more likely to end up on dialysis within the next 8 years, regardless of their starting eGFR.

Second study that demonstrates the value of BUN

Effects of blood urea nitrogen independent of the estimated glomerular filtration rate on the development of anemia in non-dialysis chronic kidney disease: The results of the KNOW-CKD study (2021)[13]

Kim HJ, Kim TE, Han MY, et al (15 authors)

Number of Patients: 2,196 with CKD in a prospective study

Results: "BUN was inversely associated with hemoglobin level. Moreover, BUN, rather than eGFR, increased the risk of anemia development in patients with CKD stage 3 in the multivariable Cox regression."

Conclusion: "Higher BUN levels derived from inappropriately high protein intake relative to renal function were associated with low hemoglobin levels and the increased risk of anemia independent of eGFR in CKD patients."

Easy-to-Read Summary: The link between high BUN and anemia showed up regardless of eGFR in kidney disease patients. This is a great example of why we have to successfully manage several factors to be successful as a kidney patient. High BUN levels contribute to low hemoglobin and anemia which is unexpected.

BUN also acts as a predictive factor for other diseases like heart disease and pneumonia.[14] A key component to building our understanding of CKD is realizing how much our kidneys and kidney-related tests like BUN affect our overall health. High BUN levels independently affect other parts of our health like anemia, hemoglobin, and how fast we head for dialysis.

Third study that shows how important BUN is for our health

Predictive value of blood urea nitrogen in heart failure: A systematic review and meta-analysis (2023)[15]

Duan S, Li Y, and Yang P (3 authors)

Number of Patients: 56,003 patients with heart failure in 19 different cohort studies around the world

Results: "When BUN was used as a variable, the risk of death in heart failure was 2.29 times higher for high levels of BUN than for low levels of BUN."

Note: For every 10 mg/dL increase in blood urea nitrogen (BUN), the mortality rate of heart failure patients increased by 21%.

Easy-to-Read-Summary: In patients with heart failure, the people with high levels of BUN died more than twice as often than people with low levels of BUN. This was statistically significant (not by chance).

Our goal is simple, we want to bring BUN levels back to the normal ranges. BUN levels in the normal ranges represent optimal levels less likely to speed kidney and heart disease progression. Again, BUN levels are on just about every blood test, so this information is easily accessible by patients and clinicians.

Creatinine is another common kidney function test, but not as predictive as GFR or BUN, so we will not cover creatinine until later in the book. Proteinuria, albuminuria, or leaking protein in your urine is also a strong predictor as are blood albumin levels. These are not reported in as many studies, so we will stick to GFR and BUN levels for now. We want to keep things simple and use tests available to every patient and clinician.

Close of Part 1

Let's go over our basic evaluation criteria for kidney diets.

We are going to evaluate kidney diets in Parts 2 and 3 based on the ability to slow disease progression (keep our GFR from falling too fast) and/or return BUN levels back to the normal ranges as objective evidence of effectiveness. Other tests or indicators could be used, but these are the big 2 in terms of accurately predicting our future outcomes that are available to every patient. **For the first time, we are going to hold these diets or dietary combinations to the same standards when no standards have existed.**

The same standards will be applied to all diets and dietary combinations in Parts 2 and 3.

A quick recap on progression rates before we continue:

- GFR loss per year greater than -7.5% represents the worst outcomes group (bottom 25%).

- GFR loss per year between -3% and -7.5% represents normal kidney disease progression and average or normal outcomes (which are not great).

- GFR loss between 0% and -3% is closer to normal age-related kidney function loss and equals better future outcomes. <u>This should be the minimum standard for kidney diets or dietary combinations.</u>

- GFR improvements greater than 0% represent the best possible outcomes, but have not been possible in the past.

For BUN, our goal is to achieve normal ranges. If BUN is 24 mg/dL or greater, then future outcomes are not as good and worsen as BUN levels rise.

Any kidney diet, supplements, foods, dietary combinations, or dietary advice can be effectively and objectively evaluated using changes in BUN and GFR. Judging our diet this way gives us an objective yardstick to guide us and help predict our future with kidney disease. This data is on almost every blood test we take.

Part 2: Established Kidney Diets: Two Groups With Two Variations

Almost every variation of kidney diet falls into 2 broad groupings as protein intake has been the primary criteria. We will go over broad groupings first, and then we will dig into a few variations of each diet and the impact of those variations.

The 2 broad groups of kidney diets are

- Low protein diets (Chapter 5)
- Very low protein diets (Chapter 6)

Subcategories of these groups addressed in this book will be

- Plant-based diets (Chapter 7)
- Protein supplementation with amino acids or keto acid analogs (Chapter 8)

<u>Please remember, the conclusions and results you are going to read are from the researchers and physicians who conducted the reviews. They are not our opinions but objective conclusions from studies.</u> I wanted to note this as many of these findings may go against current guidance depending on the source, organization, book, website, etc. This is another reason why this kind of book is desperately needed as a form of quality control for patients and clinicians.

Chapter 5

Low Protein Diets (LPD)

Low protein diets (LPD) are typically 0.6 grams to 0.8 grams of protein per kilogram of body weight per day.[1] This translates to between 47–63 g of total protein intake per day for a 175-pound (79 kg) person as a reference. The usual recommended daily amount (RDA) for protein is 0.8 g per kg of body weight, or 63 g for a 175 lb (79 kg) person. When we say total protein intake, we mean protein intake totaled for the day from all sources: diet, supplements, drinks, snacks, etc.

For comparison, normal protein intake in the US is well above 1 g of protein per kg of body weight daily. Assuming 1.2 g of protein for a more normal American diet, then a 175 lb (79 kg) person would normally consume around 95 g of protein per day. Going from 95 g of protein per day to 47 g per day for LPD is a big change in protein intake for most of us. To give you a reference, 1 cup of chopped or diced chicken contains 38 g of protein or almost 80% of the protein you are allowed to eat daily. Every food, with a handful of exceptions, contains protein, even fruits and vegetables. Broccoli florets and stalks contain 4–5 g of protein. One cup of chopped chicken with 2 florets and stalks of broccoli and you have hit your protein limit for the day on low protein diets. From a patient prescriptive, low protein diets feel like a drastic change in our diets.

Low protein diets limit protein but keep protein intake high enough so that protein supplementation should not be needed, hypothetically. Keto acid analogs or protein supplements are not used with LPD as you are meeting (or close to meeting) the RDA for protein with diet alone. This may or may not be what you choose to do, for reasons you will see later. Low protein diets may include other restrictions on sodium, potassium, phosphorus, etc.

Let's see what the largest metastudies have to say about LPD's efficacy and if LPD meets our minimum standard.

First study that describes LPD effects on kidney disease

Protein restriction for diabetic kidney disease (2023)[16]

Jiang S, Fang J, Li W (3 authors)

Number of Patients: 486 participants from 8 studies were reviewed

Results: "In low certainty evidence, a LPD may have little or no effect on death and the number of participants who reached kidney failure. Compared to a usual or unrestricted protein intake, it remains uncertain whether a LPD slows the decline of glomerular filtration rate (GFR) over time."

Easy-to-Read Summary: *Kidney disease patients who followed an LPD died and/or experienced kidney failure about as often as kidney patients on their usual diets. Both groups had similar rates of eGFR decline.*

Second study that shows minimal effect of LPD on health

Impact of low-protein diet on cardiovascular risk factors and kidney function in diabetic nephropathy: A systematic review and meta-analysis of randomized-controlled trials (2022)[17]

Sohouli MH, Mirmiran P, Seraj SS, et al (9 authors)

Number of Patients: 898 participants from 18 studies around the world between 1987–2009

Results: "The results of the present study showed that a LPD significantly reduces urinary urea and HbA1c levels. However, the results showed neither significant nor beneficial effects on other renal function and cardiovascular risk factors."

Easy-to-Read Summary: *The researchers were looking at published studies about LPDs to see what kind of effect the diet would have on heart disease risk factors and kidney function in people with diabetic kidney disease. They didn't find any important benefits in terms of kidney function or heart disease risk factors. They did find that LPD reduces urea in the urine and improves HbA1c. Urea is a waste product of protein intake, so when you reduce protein intake, urea is normally reduced by some amount.*

Third study that showed LPD and VLPD effects on health

The effects of restricted protein diet supplemented with ketoanalogue on renal function, blood pressure, nutritional status, and chronic kidney disease-mineral and bone disorder in chronic kidney disease patients: A systematic review and meta-analysis (2020)[18]

Chewcharat A, Takkavatakarn K, Wongrattanagorn S, et al (7 authors)

Number of Patients: 1,459 participants from 17 randomized controlled trials

Results: "By subgroup analysis, a very low protein diet (VLPD) with KAs [keto acid analogues] was plausibly superior to LPD with KAs in slowing the decline in eGFR. Only VLPD with KAs significantly improved serum PTH [parathyroid hormone], systolic blood pressure, and diastolic blood pressure while both regimens significantly decreased serum phosphate. Only LPD with KAs significantly raised serum albumin and serum calcium."

Conclusion: "VLPD with KAs appears to provide more effectiveness in slowing the decline in eGFR, lowering blood pressure, reducing serum PTH, and lessening serum calcium level."

Easy-to-Read Summary: *When researchers compared LPD with keto acid analogues and VLPD with keto acid analogues, they found that the diets had different effects. People on VLPDs had improved eGFR, lowered blood pressure, and improved calcium and PTH levels, but people on LPD did not show these changes. Only LPD with keto acid analogs improved albumin and calcium.*

Fourth study that showed LPD are not very effective

Efficacy of low-protein diet in diabetic nephropathy: A meta-analysis of randomized controlled trials (2018)[19]

Li XF, Xu J, Liu LJ, Wang F, He SL, Su Y, Dong CP (7 authors)

Number of Patients: 11 articles were included in the meta-analysis with a total of 1,372 patients in randomized controlled trials who met the inclusion criteria.

Results: "Moderate to strong evidence indicated that LPD was significantly effective for decreasing the urinary albumin excretion rate and proteinuria versus the control group. No statistical difference, however, was found in glycosylated hemoglobin, serum creatinine, as well as glomerular filtration rate between the two groups."

Easy-to-Read Summary: *Protein in urine was reduced due to lower protein intake. However, GFR, hemoglobin A1c, and creatinine levels did not improve using a low protein diet.*

Fifth study showing lack of effect of LPD and effectiveness of VLPD

Low protein diets for non-diabetic adults with chronic kidney disease (2020)[20]

Hahn D, Hodson EM, Fouque D (3 authors)

Number of patients: 2996 participants from 17 studies with nondiabetic CKD 3–5

Conclusion: "This review found that very low protein diets probably reduce the number of people with CKD 4 or 5 who progress to ESKD. In contrast, low protein diets may make little difference to the number of people who progress to ESKD.

Easy-to-Read Summary: *The review found that following an LPD doesn't help people with CKD 4 or 5 from ending up on dialysis. However, a VLPD does delay the start of dialysis by slowing kidney disease progression.*

What is most interesting about this last study is that it was originally published in 2000 and then updated in 2006, 2009, 2018, and then again in 2020. The conclusions changed from the original study (2000) which suggested that reducing protein intake by 40% reduced the number of patients going to dialysis, or basically, a form of low protein diets (LPD) showed promise. However, by 2020 the conclusion was that low protein diets (LPD) do not make a difference, but VLPD+KA diets do. This is a great example of researchers updating conclusions as more data became available. What was recommended in 2000 is no longer recommended 20 years later in 2020, and the guidance is more precise.

Sixth study on low protein diets

Low-protein diet for conservative management of chronic kidney disease: A systematic review and meta-analysis of controlled trials (2018)[21]

Rhee CM, Ahmadi SF, Kovesdy CP, Kalantar-Zadeh K (4 authors)

Number of patients: 2,771 with CKD 3–5, some with diabetes, from 16 different RCTs

Results: "Compared with diets with protein intake of >0.8 g/kg/day, diets with restricted protein intake (<0.8 g/kg/day) were associated with higher serum bicarbonate levels, lower phosphorus levels, lower azotemia, lower rates of progression to end-stage renal disease, and a trend towards lower rates of all-cause death. In addition, very-low-protein diets (protein intake <0.4 g/kg/day) were associated with greater preservation of kidney function and reduction in the rate of progression to end-stage renal disease."

Easy-to-Read Summary: People who followed LPD had better numbers on their blood tests, were less likely to need dialysis, and were somewhat less likely to die from any cause. People who followed a VLPD had the above benefits, plus their kidney function was more likely to be preserved (not get worse). The people on LPD and VLPD did not have increased malnutrition rates.

What do 6 metastudies and systematic reviews from 2006–2023 tell us about low protein diets and kidney disease progression?

Let's work out the facts from 10,000+ patients, 80+ individual studies, and the opinions of 30+ physicians published in peer-reviewed journals. This is very, very high-quality evidence.

Evidence based on GFR/eGFR and BUN levels

1. GFR or eGFR loss averaged > -7.5% decline for LPD as a group. LPD diets put us in the bottom 25% of future outcomes.

2. Blood urea nitrogen (BUN) levels continued to rise on LPD with no studies reporting a decline in blood urea nitrogen levels. No study reported achieving normal BUN levels.

3. No study suggested or found that low protein diets slow kidney disease progression. All 6 meta-analyses agree, there are no conflicting opinions spanning 10,000+ patients and over 30 physicians/researchers.

Other relevant data for us to consider

1. Based on what we know about kidney function and waste products, any amount of protein restriction may be beneficial, but eating 0.6 g of protein per kg of body weight per day or more puts us in the worst outcomes group or bottom 25% of future outcomes. GFR continued to drop quickly, and BUN did not normalize.

2. LPD are expected to provide enough daily protein intake without protein supplements. However, albumin (the most common protein in our bloodstream) only improved on LPD when supplemented with keto acid analogs. The implication is LPD are not providing enough nutrition on their own or keto acid analogs are providing other benefits not provided by LPD alone. Either way, LPD are more deficient than previously thought. Albumin is very difficult to raise, so this is noteworthy.

3. 2024 KDIGO[2] no longer recommends low protein diets (LPD) stating:

   "The Work Group considers that the evidence does not support a recommendation to follow low-protein diets alone as a strategy to slow the progression of CKD."

4. The 2020 KDOQI[1] does recommend low protein diets (LPD) which is a conflicting recommendation compared to the 2024 KDIGO recommendation. The wording in the 2020 KDOQI also implies that low protein diets (LPD) are as effective as very low protein diets with keto acid analogs (VLPD+KA), which is not correct as you will see in the next chapter.

When we talk about the need for objective standards, transparency, disclosure, best practices, proven effectiveness and up-to-date information, low protein diets are the poster child of why this is so important to our future outcomes.

When 2 simple standards (GFR trajectory or trend and normal BUN levels) are applied, we find there is no evidence that LPD are effective in slowing or managing kidney disease. No one disagrees with these findings, yet low protein diets (LPD) are still a commonly recommended kidney diet today.[22]

In 2025, tens of thousands of kidney patients follow plans or diets with no evidence of effectiveness. This year, new kidney diet books, websites and many clinicians are still advocating low protein diets or even higher protein diets despite all evidence to the contrary. I can't emphasize enough how big a problem this is for us as a patient group. LPD was advocated in the 1980s and early 1990s, thus representing 30–40-year-old recommendations that still persist today. Again, your education is the best form of self-defense, and education is the best way to advocate for yourself or a family member.

Other reviewers came to the same conclusion in 2022,[17,23] stating that LPD has no proof of effectiveness and should no longer be recommended.

When we don't have an objective standard or yardstick to measure effectiveness (like prescription drugs do), then anything can be said to be effective or ineffective. The lack of an objective standard has allowed the least effective dietary advice with the most available evidence to become the most common. If you wanted evidence that unregulated and unproven dietary advice is hurting us as a patient group, here it is.

In 2025, there is no confusion or debate regarding the lack of effectiveness of low protein diets.

From a patient perspective, low protein diets are as much work as any other kidney diet, but they don't have any measurable benefits and may have nutritional shortfalls as well.

Please go over the data in this chapter with anyone recommending a low protein diet and fully discuss the implications for your future health and what is best for you.

Chapter 6

Very Low Protein Diets With Keto Acid Analogs (VLPD+KA)

These diets normally restrict protein by 50% more than LPD by using 0.3–0.4 g of dietary protein per kg of body weight per day. It is confusing as *very low protein diets* sound exactly like *low protein diets*, but adding the word *very* represents a 50% reduction in protein intake.

Using the same 175-lb (79 kg) person from last chapter as an example, daily dietary protein intake would be between 23–31 g per day from diet. These diets are always supplemented with keto acid analogs in some manner to avoid protein malnutrition as protein intake from food is always below the RDA. Using the example from the LPD chapter, VLPD protein restriction would be ½ cup of chicken and 1 floret and stalk of broccoli for the day. This is an important issue because when we drop below 0.3 g/kg of dietary protein intake, these diets become impossible in real life. A 0.3 g/kg protein restriction should be considered the absolute floor for dietary protein restriction. A 0.3 g/kg protein restriction is a very tough restriction but it is possible. This is an important fact when judging effectiveness because if we cannot hit our goals with .3 g/kg dietary protein restriction then we are at the end of the dietary road. We will have to use another approach.

The primary purpose of lowering protein intake and using keto acid analogs instead is to reduce the problems from high BUN levels. Other benefits also exist like lowering phosphorus and renal acid load. In the past, lowering BUN levels has been the primary goal.

Can lowering dietary protein intake by 50% and adding keto acid analogs slow disease progression compared to low protein diets (LPD)? Can we change the slope of kidney disease progression or bring BUN levels back to normal?

Five large reviews/studies were available for VLPDs. A few of these were also covered in the LPD chapter. I will list these studies again so you don't have to page back and forth.

First study showing effects of keto acids on LPD and VLPD

Effect of restricted protein diet supplemented with keto analogues in chronic kidney disease: A systematic review and meta-analysis (2016)[24]

Jiang Z, Zhang X, Yang L, Li Z, Qin W (5 authors)

Number of Patients: 410 with CKD 3–5 from 7 random control trials, 1 cross-over trial and 1 non-randomized concurrent control trial

Results: "The meta-analysis results indicated that, compared with normal protein diet, low protein diet (LPD) or very low protein diet (vLPD) supplemented with keto analogues could significantly prevent the deterioration of eGFR, hyperparathyroidism, hypertension, and hyperphosphatemia. No differences in BUN, creatinine, albumin, triglyceride, cholesterol, hemoglobin, calcium and nutrition indexes were observed between different protein intake groups."

Conclusion: "Restricted protein diet supplemented with keto analogues could delay the progression of CKD effectively without causing malnutrition."

Easy-to-Read Summary: The researchers looked at groups of people who ate normal diets, LPDs, and VLPDs. The people who limited the amount of protein in the diet had better kidney function (eGFR) and lower rates of certain other problems (hyperparathyroidism, high blood pressure, high blood phosphate). Limiting protein in the diet didn't help with every problem—blood tests for anemia, BUN, creatinine, cholesterol, calcium, and albumin (protein) were about the same.

Second study that showed effects of KA on protein restricted diets

The effects of restricted protein diet supplemented with ketoanalogue on renal function, blood pressure, nutritional status, and chronic kidney disease-mineral and bone disorder in chronic kidney disease patients: A systematic review and meta-analysis (2020)[18]

Chewcharat A, Takkavatakarn K, Wongrattanagorn S, et al (7 authors)

Number of Patients: 1,459 participants from 17 randomized controlled trials

Results: "By subgroup analysis, a very low protein diet (VLPD) with KAs was plausibly superior to LPD with KAs in slowing the decline in eGFR. Only VLPD with KAs significantly improved serum PTH, systolic blood pressure, and diastolic blood pressure while both regimens significantly decreased serum phosphate. Only LPD with KAs significantly raised serum albumin and serum calcium."

Conclusion: "Restricted protein diet supplemented with KAs could effectively improve kidney endpoints, including preserving eGFR and diminishing proteinuria, blood pressure levels, and CKD-mineral bone disorder parameters without causing malnutrition. VLPD with KAs appears to provide more effectiveness in slowing the decline in eGFR, lowering blood pressure, reducing serum PTH, and lessening serum calcium level."

Easy-to-Read Summary: When researchers compared LPD with keto acid analogues and VLPD with keto acid analogues, they found that the diets had different effects. People on VLPDs had improved eGFR, lowered blood pressure, and improved calcium and PTH levels.

Third study comparing LPD and VLPD

Low-protein diet for conservative management of chronic kidney disease: A systematic review and meta-analysis of controlled trials (2018)[19]

Rhee CM, Ahmadi SF, Kovesdy CP, Kalantar-Zadeh K (4 authors)

Number of Patients: 2,771 with CKD 3–5, some with diabetes, from 16 different RCTs

Results: "Compared with diets with protein intake of >0.8 g/kg/day, diets with restricted protein intake (<0.8 g/kg/day) were associated with higher serum bicarbonate levels, lower phosphorus levels, lower azotemia, lower rates of progression to end-stage renal disease, and a trend towards lower rates of all-cause death. In addition, very-low-protein diets (protein intake <0.4 g/kg/day) were associated with greater preservation of kidney function and reduction in the rate of progression to end-stage renal disease."

Easy-to-Read Summary: People who followed LPD had better numbers on their blood tests, were less likely to need dialysis, and were less likely to die from any cause. People who followed a VLPD had the above benefits, plus their kidney function was more likely to be preserved (not get worse). The people on LPD and VLPD did not have increased malnutrition rates.

Fourth study showing positive effects on CKD using VLPD

Low protein diets for non-diabetic adults with chronic kidney disease (2020)[20]

Hahn D, Hodson EM, Fouque D (3 authors)

Number of Patients: 2,996 participants from 17 studies with nondiabetic CKD 3–5.

Conclusion: "This review found that very low protein diets probably reduce the number of people with CKD 4 or 5 who progress to ESKD. In contrast, low protein diets may make little difference to the number of people who progress to ESKD."

Easy-to-Read Summary: *The review found that following an LPD doesn't help people with CKD 4 or 5 from ending up on dialysis or needing a kidney transplant. However, a VLPD does keep people off of or delay dialysis.*

Fifth study showing the effects of VLPD with KA on CKD

The effect of the diet of nitrogen-free analogs of essential amino acids on chronic kidney disease deterioration: A meta-analysis (2022)[25]

Yang W (1 author)

Number of Patients: 1574 CKD patients from 14 studies

Results: "Very low-protein diet supplemented with nitrogen-free analogs had significantly higher estimated glomerular filtration rate, lower serum creatinine, and lower blood urea nitrogen; however, it had no significant difference in serum albumin, serum cholesterol, serum phosphorus, serum calcium, and parathyroid hormone compared to conventional low-protein diet in subjects with chronic kidney disease."

Conclusion: "The very low-protein diets supplemented with nitrogen-free analogs had significantly better kidney functions results compared to the conventional low-protein diets in subjects with chronic kidney disease."

Easy-to-Read Summary: *VLPD with low nitrogen keto acid analogues improved lab values like eGFR, creatinine, and BUN compared to LPD. This means that kidney function is improved in VLPD compared to LPD. However, not everything was improved—protein (albumin), cholesterol, and labs for parathyroid disease (PTH, calcium, phosphorus)—were the same for both LPD and VLPD.*

Unpacking the key findings

20+ physicians using data from 9,000+ patients and 50+ studies concluded that VLPD+KA preserved kidney function or improved the trajectory of GFR better than LPDs. Again, we have excellent evidence just like low protein diet studies.

Evidence based on GFR/eGFR and BUN levels

1. Unfortunately, disease progression with a VLPD+KA still falls within the normal ranges of kidney disease progression, but we are no longer in the worst outcomes group. GFR loss averaged -4.5% a year for VLPD as a group. We are now in the average outcomes group, a step up from the worst outcomes group using LPD of -7.5 % or greater annual loss. We have gone from the worst case (on LPD or regular diet) to more normal progression with VLPD. This is still not the best-case scenario we are after, but is an improvement for us if we compare it to LPD.

2. Normal BUN levels were not achieved by any study. BUN levels did drop by an average of -20.1% on VLPD+KA which is noteworthy and valuable, but normal ranges were not attained. In contrast, BUN levels rose on LPD.

3. No conflicting opinions exist. All studies found that VLPD+KA diets slowed the loss of kidney disease progression by some amount and were superior compared to LPD.

Other relevant information from these studies

1. Very low protein diets with keto acid analogs (VLPD+KA) are recommended by both the 2020 KDOQI[1] and the 2024 KDIGO.[2] Both agree VLPD+KA have enough evidence to recommend broadly. This is important to us, as we find 2 reputable organizations agreeing on the same approach. This kind of agreement is noteworthy as a form of quality control.

2. We changed 2 things with VLPD+KA. We lowered protein intake by 50% and added keto acid analogs for protein supplementation. Was it diet, keto acid analogs, or the combination that improved results? We cannot determine this from VLPD+KA studies, but we will attempt to answer this question in the chapter on keto acid analogs (Chapter 8).

3. No combination of 0.3 g/kg/day protein restriction with nitrogen content from keto acid analogs between 450–860 mg achieved normal BUN levels. This is important as we cannot go lower than a 0.3 g/kg/day dietary protein restriction in real life. This tells us that normal BUN levels cannot be achieved using past combinations of traditional keto acid analogs and very low protein diets. It's important to understand this fact when evaluating online claims.

Summary

Slowing disease progression by 25%–40% by switching from LPD to VLPD+KA has the potential to add years of useful life to our kidneys. This is not a small amount and the difference between the 2 diets was a clinically significant change or outcome.

While no confusion exists on LPD vs VLPD+KA in terms of effectiveness thanks to head-to-head studies, confusion does exist when you compare VLPD+KA to normal rates of kidney disease progression. It's not really clear if VLPD works or not, unless you compare them to a worse dietary combination (low protein diets) or very fast kidney disease progression.

We are moving in a much better direction with VLPD+KA, but we still not quite achieving our real goals of slowing progression to rates slower than normal disease progression rates or achieving normal BUN levels.

Please go over the data in this chapter with any clinicians or professionals recommending a VLPD+KA dietary approach to determine what is right for you and if you can achieve your goals using this approach.

Chapter 7

Plant-Based Diets for Kidney Disease

Section 1: The Evidence on Plant-Based

The single most common call/email we get is something like "I don't understand, I went plant-based, vegan, or vegetarian, and I am not improving!" This topic needs a full chapter to discuss due to the sheer number of questions we receive. If the number of emails and calls is an accurate representation of patient confusion, then plant-based diets are the most confusing dietary approach to kidney disease.

The perception that plant-based diets solve every problem is due to the marketing of plant-based diets combined with modern medical guidance recommending plant-based, Mediterranean diets and increased fruit and vegetable intake. These diets may also be referred to as PLADO diets which stands for *plant-dominant low-protein diets*. Everyone's assumption (and I mean everyone's) is that plant-based diets help us with kidney disease progression without looking at the evidence first. There are lots of facts on plant-based diets, but there are also lots of myths and misconceptions that we need to correct. Almost all research on kidney disease and plant based diets is theoretical. Authors theorize about the potential benefits of plant based diets for kidney patients. There is nothing wrong with this, but we are going to focus on studies with humans, not theories. When we eliminate theoretical studies, we get a much clearer picture on plant based diets.

Plant-based diets do have the most promise, but they also have the most pitfalls. In other words, it's easier to screw up a plant-based diet than any other diet because of all of the specialized issues that have to be dealt with successfully. I will do my best to break out each individual issue in a clear, concise way.

Let's start with big-picture reviews and studies.

Four large-scale reviews exist to start us off, but I am breaking out each study in the first review as the data is very educational on specific diets and the effects on kidney disease progression, which we know is what matters to us patients—slowing disease progression means delaying dialysis or transplant.

The impact of a vegetarian diet on chronic kidney disease (CKD) progression – a systematic review (2023)[26]

Świątek Ł, Jeske J, Miedziaszczyk M, Idasiak-Piechocka I (4 authors)

Number of Patients: 346 participants from 4 trials

Results: "Two largest RCTs [randomized controlled trials] reported an increase in eGFR following a change to a vegetarian diet ($p = 0.01$ and $p = 0.001$). Another two found no significant differences between the experimental and control groups, also these trials were associated with a high risk of bias."

Easy-to-Read Summary: Of the 4 studies they reviewed, the largest 2 studies showed that people had a statistically significant improvement in eGFR after switching to a vegetarian diet (meaning the effect was not due to chance). The other 2 didn't show effects, but they weren't as large or well-designed.

Now let's look at the individual studies within this review for a better understanding of the issues here. We started with a 50/50 chance of benefits (2 of 4 showed a benefit). From a drug standard, a 50/50 chance of improvement would doom any drug to failure.

Comparison 1 (from a paper titled "Effects of vegetarian versus Mediterranean diet on kidney function: Findings from the CARDIVEG study"[27])

Diets compared	Starting GFR	Ending GFR
Lacto-ovo vegetarian[3]	96.5	99
Mediterranean diets	97	95.7

If your GFR is over 90, vegetarian diets improve GFR by 2.5 points or around 2.5% (a very small amount). The original researchers were interested in heart disease, not kidney disease, so they didn't select patients with CKD.[27]

Comparison 2 (from a paper titled "Ketoanalogue-supplemented vegetarian very low-protein diet and CKD progression"[28])

Diets	Starting GFR	Ending GFR
Vegetarian VLPD+KA	18	15.1
LPD	17.9	10.8

---

3   Lacto-ovo vegetarians eat dairy (lacto) and eggs (ovo) as well as vegetables, fruits, legumes, and nuts.

Disease progression was slowed meaningfully using plant-based VLPD+KA compared with LPD, which is the same as we witnessed in chapters on LPD (Chapter 5) and VLPD+KA (Chapter 6). The finding here is that plant-based diets must also be very low in protein (0.3 g/kg of protein per day was used in this study) and use keto acid analogs to be effective. It's also true that GFR numbers dropped meaningfully on both diets, and normal BUN levels were not achieved.

Comparison 3 (from a paper titled "Withdrawal of red meat from the usual diet reduces albuminuria and improves serum fatty acid profile in Type 2 diabetes patients with macroalbuminuria"[29])

Diets	Starting GFR	Ending GFR
Usual diets	81.8	81.8
Protein limited to chicken	81.8	83.3
Lacto-vegetarian diet	81.8	81.9

The same patients switched to different diets and results were measured, so the starting GFR is the same. This study also wasn't designed with CKD patients in mind.[29] Lacto-vegetarian diets are vegetarian diets that allow dairy products to be consumed.

Comparison 4 (from a paper titled "Comparison of a vegetable-based (soya) and an animal-based low-protein diet in predialysis chronic renal failure patients"[30])

Diets	Starting GFR	Ending GFR
LPD vegetarian diet	28.8	28.1
LPD with animal-based protein	28.8	29.6

The same patients switched diets like the previous study, so we see the same starting GFR numbers. In this case, the plant-based diet was slightly worse than the animal-protein-based diet despite the same protein intake.

Perceptions versus outcomes

To drive a point home about dietary perceptions and actual outcomes, let's list the different diets from this study and look at results to see if normal BUN levels were achieved or if GFR was slowed to a rate slower than normal disease progression rates.

Diet type	Achieve normal BUN	Improve GFR
Usual	No	No
Protein limited to chicken	No	No
Lacto-vegetarian	No	No
VLPD+KA plant-based	No	No
Mediterranean	No	No
LPD vegetarian	No	No
LPD with animal protein	No	No

The perception from both patients and clinicians is that they made a big dietary change that was going to make a measurable difference in outcomes. However, no published evidence exists that any of these dietary combinations improve anything except for plant-based VLPD+KA. Plant-based VLPD+KA reduced BUN levels, but not back to the normal range. **The lesson is our dietary perceptions are normally wrong, very wrong compared with dietary reality. Do not make any assumptions without seeing the evidence first.**

Second study showing the effects of plant-based protein on CKD

Effects of plant-based protein consumption on kidney function and mineral bone disorder outcomes in adults with stage 3-5 chronic kidney disease: A systematic review (2023)[31]

Burstad KM, Cladis DP, Wiese GN, Butler M, Gallant KMH (5 authors)

Number of Patients: 1182 patients with CKD 3–5 from 32 different studies

Discussion: "Of the subset of five studies where a change in protein source from animal to plant-based protein was the main intervention, short or mid-length duration studies showed no change in kidney function… Indeed, the long-term study by Barsotti et al was the only study to report a change in kidney function with a vegetarian low-protein diet, but the change observed was a worsening rather than an improvement of kidney function."

Easy-to-Read Summary: *Of the 32 studies that tried to answer questions about kidney function and protein, most of them weren't designed to directly answer whether vegetarian diets or meat-based diets were better. So, the researchers chose the 5 studies which did directly compare plant- and animal-based diets. Of those 5 studies, 4 of them didn't show any real changes in eGFR. The 1 study that did show a change in eGFR showed that a vegetarian LPD had worse outcomes.*

Third study showing comparison of vegetarian diets for CKD patients

Effect of vegetarian diets on renal function in patients with chronic kidney disease under non-dialysis treatment: A scoping review (2022)[32]

Valim A, Carpes LS, Nicoletto BB (3 authors)

Number of Patients: 324 patients with CKD 3–5 from 4 studies

Abstract: "One study showed that <u>a very low-protein ketoanalogue-supplemented vegetarian diet had benefits in relation to a conventional low-protein diet, while the other three studies demonstrated no difference in kidney function between the evaluated diets.</u>"

Easy-to-Read Summary: *Only 1 type of very low protein (0.3 g/kg) vegetarian diet with keto acid analogs had measurable benefits. Other variations of vegetarian diets demonstrated no effect on kidney function.*

Fourth study on plant-based diets and kidney disease progression

Adherence to plant-based diets and risk of CKD progression and all-cause mortality: Findings from the chronic renal insufficiency cohort (CRIC) study (2023)[33]

Amir S, Kim H, Hu EA, et al. (14 authors)

Number of Patients: 2,539 participants with CKD

Discussion: In conclusion, higher adherence to an overall plant-based diet and a healthy plant-based diet was associated with a reduced risk of all-cause mortality but not CKD progression or incident cardiovascular disease in a population of kidney disease patients. However, unhealthy plant-based diets were linked to faster kidney disease progression.

Easy-to-Read Summary: *Plant-based diets lowered the mortality (death) rate for kidney patients over both 7-year and 12-year measurement periods, but plant-based diets had no measurable effect on kidney disease progression or heart disease. Unhealthy plant-based diets did increase the speed of kidney disease progression. If we get plant-based diets right, disease progression is not slowed, but if we get these diets wrong, then kidney disease progression may speed up.*

What are unhealthy plant-based diets and ultra processed foods?

I feel the need to cover these topics here before continuing as the study above brought up the concepts of *unhealthy plant-based diets* and *ultra-processed foods*.

The CRIC study on plant based diets noted the following associations with unhealthy plant-based diets and faster disease progression:

1. "Unhealthy plant-based diets were high in refined grains, potatoes, fruit juices, sugar-sweetened beverages, sweets, and desserts, and low in healthy plant foods and animal foods, which resulted in low fiber and micronutrient intake.

2. "In our study, consumption of sugar-sweetened beverages was significantly associated with all-cause mortality, whereas higher fiber intake was associated with a lower risk of CKD progression and all-cause mortality.

3. "Previous studies have linked unhealthy plant-based diets to adverse health outcomes, including incident diabetes, hypertension, and coronary heart disease

4. "In the CRIC cohort, greater consumption of ultra processed foods was associated with a higher risk of all-cause mortality and CKD progression.

5. "Taken together, our findings provide support for reducing consumption of unhealthy plant foods, such as sugar-sweetened beverages, and increasing consumption of fiber-rich foods to lower the risk of CKD progression."

What are ultra processed foods?

While no standard definitions exist, ultra-processed foods are normally defined as manufactured foods with 3 ingredients or more. Five ingredients might be a more realistic definition. Ultra-processed foods are made from combinations of manufactured ingredients. Many plant-based products made to taste and look like meat have 20+ ingredients. As an example, the number one ingredient in plant-based chicken nuggets is normally flour. These manufactured ingredients are typically lower in nutrition, fiber, antioxidants, etc. when compared to whole foods. The theme for ultra-processed foods is higher calorie and lower nutrition. The lesson is just because something is plant-based, vegan, or vegetarian doesn't mean it's healthy for us.

Nutritional profiles change with ultra-processed foods

Pea protein is a good example. Many patients assume products like pea protein (or any other plant-based protein) are just ground up or powdered peas. However, all plant-based protein powders go through a manufacturing or extraction process to remove the fiber and starch which also removes or reduces many of the micronutrients and antioxidants present in peas. The nutritional profile of pea protein is completely different from real peas. These products are designed to be very high in amino acids (protein) and low in everything else. We get all the bad stuff (high-nitrogen amino acids) and very little of the good (fiber, antioxidants, vitamins, etc.). These kinds of plant(or animal) based protein bars, powders, drinks etc.. are normally a very poor choice for kidney patients, see the chapter on amino acids to better understand why. (Chapter 8)

Our lesson is that manufactured or ultra processed foods are a completely different food by design and have completely different nutritional values despite being plant based.

Let's unpack what we can from studies.

Over 40 studies, 4,300+ patients, and 26 researchers/physicians found no evidence that changing from animal-based to plant-based protein or changing to a plant-based diet changes the trajectory of kidney disease or achieves normal BUN levels.

Evidence based on GFR/eGFR and BUN levels and other relevant information

1. No improvement in GFR was documented using different variations of plant-based diets alone for actual kidney patients (GFR below 60). GFR did drop less on a plant-based VLPD+KA diet, but the plant-based diet had to be very low in protein and supplemented with keto acid analogs. Plant-based diets alone have no published record of success in slowing kidney disease progression.

2. BUN was not measured in most of these studies, so we can't comment in detail. The studies that did report BUN levels did not return BUN levels back to normal. Plant based diets alone have no published record of achieving normal BUN levels.

3. The 2020 KDOQI[1] stated that no difference could be demonstrated between animal and plant proteins.

When you combine these studies with the 2020 KDOQI conclusion that no difference could be demonstrated between animal- and plant-based proteins,[1] you have very strong evidence that going plant-based, vegan, or vegetarian alone has little-to-no evidence of effectiveness.

To be crystal clear and reduce confusion, not a single published study exists suggesting plant-based diets alone slow kidney disease progression to rates slower than normal kidney disease progression or achieve normal BUN levels, not one. However, you can speed up kidney disease progression with unhealthy plant-based diets.

There are numerous studies theorizing about the potential benefits of plant based diets on kidney disease progression, but these are all theoretical, not actually proven in kidney patients. This is a very important distinction for us to be aware of in terms of quality control and guardrails.

It is possible and likely that some aspects of your blood or urine tests will improve on plant-based diets. The catch is these improvements are normally pretty minor in nature and likely don't change our future outcomes. If you are measuring GFR trajectories and BUN levels, then no benefit could be found. Applying these objective standards cleared things up immediately. Plant-based diets are marketed heavily to kidney patients despite all evidence to the contrary.

Six individual studies showed that plant-based kidney diets were not superior to animal-based diets when compared head-to-head.

Section 2 The rest of the story on plant-based diets

Plant-based diets alone have insurmountable obstacles

Again, I want to clearly explain why plant-based diets have problems because it is the most common question we get.

Let's start with a look at the change in protein intake when we switch diets.[34]

Type of diet	Average protein intake per day
Meat-based diets	90 g
Vegetarian	71 g
Vegan	64 g
Low protein diet (LPD)	60 g
Very low protein diet (VLPD)	**30 g**

If you switch from a meat-based diet with 90+ g of protein per day to a plant-based diet of 64–71 g of protein per day, your numbers may improve slightly because your overall protein intake is reduced. While going plant-based is effective in reducing the overall protein intake to some extent, the problem is the protein intake is still too high to slow disease progression rates. This is one of the primary reasons plant-based diets have been unable to show a benefit. Protein intake must be much lower for any diet to show a measurable benefit. We know factually from the LPD chapter that protein intake of 0.6 g/kg was 100% unsuccessful.

The implication is clear: it is the amount of protein that matters, not the source of the protein (plant or animal). Let me explain using basic chemistry.

Basic chemistry proves what we see in studies

The chemical makeup of every amino acid is identical whether the amino acid is plant- or animal-based. For example, the amino acid leucine from animal-based foods is chemically and nutritionally 100% identical to leucine in plant-based foods including nitrogen content. This means when we match protein amounts (60 g animal-based vs 60 g plant-based protein) we get a similar waste workload on our kidneys. This is one of the reasons why plant-based diets have not been able to show a benefit in many studies. Nothing really changed in terms of waste workload despite the perception that a major change in diet was made.

Using USDA data, let's compare a 100-gram serving of tofu[35] vs a 100-gram hamburger patty (3.5 oz) as an example.

Amino Acids

Food #	Hamburger patty	Tofu
Weight (g)	100	100
Histidine (mg)	402	431
Isoleucine (mg)	642	849
Leucine (mg)	1130	1392
Lysine (mg)	785	883
Methionine (mg)	306	211
Phenylalanine (mg)	670	835
Threonine (mg)	460	785
Tryptophan (mg)	144	235
Valine (mg)	728	870
Arginine (mg)	852	1369
Cystine (mg)	57	0
Glycine (mg)	891	733
Proline (mg)	1666	1084
Tyrosine (mg)	373	701
Alanine (mg)	785	773
Aspartic acid (mg)	1054	2036

Glutamic acid (mg)	3639	3288
Hydroxyproline (mg)	240	0
Serine (mg)	632	1015
Total amino acids (mg)	**15,499**	**17,647**
Estimated nitrogen content (mg)	**2,324**	**2,647**

Each amino acid on this list is chemically and nutritionally identical, regardless of source (tofu vs beef). A hamburger patty may actually have lower nitrogen content than a similar serving size of tofu because it has fewer amino acids. This means your blood urea nitrogen (BUN) numbers will hypothetically get slightly worse using tofu instead of a hamburger patty in this example. Making things even more complicated is that different databases show different amounts of amino acids depending on types or brands adding to confusion and uncertainty.

The takeaway is that plant-based proteins (amino acids) are not somehow magically different from animal-based proteins. They are identical in terms of waste workload on our kidneys. This should end much of this debate.

Benefits of plant-based diets with a catch

On the other hand, plant-based diets do contain more fiber and antioxidants, offer less saturated fat, lower acid load, lower phosphorus, and provide lots of other well-known benefits.[36] You could make the argument that these benefits make plant-based diets worthwhile, but what is the point of going vegan, vegetarian, or plant-based if our kidney function is declining rapidly or still progressing at normal rates? As we discussed, no published evidence exists, only theories about the potential benefits of plant based diets. We have to ask these kinds of questions as patients. There always seems to be a catch.

The VLPD+KA plant-based diet that showed a benefit in terms of slowing disease progression was tested a second time by a different group with slightly different restrictions, yet the second trial did not duplicate the outcome.[37] For this reason, we still have an open question on very low protein plant-based diets.

In terms of protein nutrition, we have to solve another problem.

Data suggests we cannot get the RDAs met for essential amino acids with intake of less than 0.7 g/kg of protein per day on plant-based diets.

Plant-based protein daily limit	Meets RDAs for EAAs?
0.8 g of protein	Yes
0.7 g of protein	Yes
0.6 g of protein	No
0.5 g of protein	No

EAA = Essential Amino Acids

Here's one study that examines this problem with a computer model.

Nutritional adequacy of animal-based and plant-based Asian diets for chronic kidney disease patients: A modeling study (2021)[38]

Khor BH, Tallman DA, Karupaiah T, Khosla P, Chan M, Kopple JD (6 authors)

Number of Patients: 0 (this was a theoretical study done with a computer program)

Conclusions: "Our food pattern modeling indicated that the Asian plant-based and vegetarian diets providing 0.7 g protein/kg/day or more could meet the RDA for all EAAs. However, at the protein prescription of 0.6 g/kg/day, only the conventional diet consisting of 50% high biological protein from animal-based foods is able to meet the RDA of all EAAs, while the vegetarian or plant-based LPDs are likely to be deficient in EAAs. Therefore, a higher protein level (at least 0.7 g protein/kg/day) should be considered for individuals who wish to adhere to vegetarian or plant-based diets, and these diets must be carefully planned because the protein prescription is still below the RDA."

Easy-to-Read Summary: The researchers used a computer to test the amounts of each essential amino acid found in different low protein diets. They found that the less overall protein in the diet, the more careful they had to be about selecting foods. At 0.7 g/kg/day, all diets provided enough essential amino acids. Between 0.5–0.7 g/kg/day, only animal-based diets included enough essential amino acids. They advised that all LPD require careful planning.

This study was on typical Asian diets, but the calculations are within 8% of our own calculations for the typical American equivalent.

Plant-based diets have a protein problem.

The inescapable dilemma for plant-based diets is that raising the protein intake to levels high enough to meet the RDAs for each essential amino acid effectively dooms these dietary programs to failure in terms of slowing GFR decline or achieving normal BUN levels. Essential amino acid nutrition varies widely from one plant-based food to another, so it's very difficult, if not impossible to get 100% of the RDAs for the 9 essential amino acids and to limit protein intake at the same time on a plant-based diet. If we don't raise protein intake high enough, then we risk protein malnutrition issues which are a real concern.

In chapter 5, it was well documented that dietary protein intake greater than .6 g/kg of body weight(LPD) put us in the worst outcomes group, losing more than -7.5% in GFR points per year. Plant based diets are clearly not exempt from this rule. Studies report similar results with plant based diets with protein intake with .6 g/kg or higher. LPD plant based diets have almost identical outcomes to LPD diets because intake is largely the same despite wearing a label of plant based. When we add the data from the LPD chapter and the plant based chapter, we cover 120 studies of 14,300 patients and the conclusions of 56 researchers and physicians. In summary, plant based diets are normally LPD diets in disguise. Plant-based diets are absolutely healthier overall for normal, healthy patients and have great potential to be beneficial to us. However, these diets have to be heavily, heavily modified and supplemented with keto acid analogs to have any potential for us kidney patients.

Whether a diet is vegan, vegetarian, or plant-based appears to be a completely irrelevant detail if you are judging the diet based on kidney disease progression rates or achieving normal BUN levels.

Plant based diets are marketed heavily to kidney patients in 2025 despite a complete lack of real world evidence. I will keep saying, "your education is your guard rail".

Please go over this chapter with any company or person advocating you change to a plant-based diet with daily protein intake at 0.6 g per kg of body weight or higher before making any decisions. If you go below 0.7 g/kg for daily protein, then some form of protein supplementation is required to ensure RDAs for protein are met.

Chapter 8

Protein Supplementation (Keto Acid Analogs and Amino Acids)

Section 1: The Evidence on Keto Acids

Now that we have covered the basic diets and one variation, we need to dig into one last common feature in kidney diets to complete our basic education.

A key component of very low protein diets (VLPD) is the use of keto acid analogs or keto acid analogues or keto acids, referred to as KA. Keto acid analog use is widely misunderstood, so it needs a chapter to explain the issue. Based on 2025 evidence, KA appears to be part of the building blocks of successful kidney diets.

VLPD always uses keto acid analogs to supplement protein intake as VLPD do not supply the RDA for proteins. It can be difficult to determine if keto acid analogs alone benefit these patients. We don't know if it's the diet, the keto acid analogs, or the combination providing the benefit.

In an effort to tease out any beneficial effects of keto acid analogs alone, we will take an alternative approach and not cover VLPD+KA in this chapter. This has been covered in Chapter 6 and would not yield any new or useful information.

Instead, we will cover results when low protein diets (LPD) are supplemented with keto acid analogs and look for head-to-head studies to get a more informed, objective opinion. I will also cover amino acid use as we get so many questions on this issue.

Let's review what keto acids analogs are again, as this is a new concept to most.

Essential amino acids are the nine amino acids our bodies cannot make. These essential amino acids are what we think of as "protein". A low protein food is low in amino acids, a high protein food is high in amino acids. We must get these amino acids from dietary intake. All amino acids contain nitrogen, which must be removed so our bodies can use nitrogen-free versions of amino acids. When the nitrogen component is removed, these amino acids are now considered keto acid analogs. Keto acid analogs are simply essential amino acids with the nitrogen waste component removed. This removal happens in the body all the time. For example, before your body can use the amino acid leucine, it needs to remove the nitrogen component and convert it to the keto acid analog of leucine first. Our bodies do this removal and send the nitrogen waste products to our kidneys for excretion. You see these waste products in bloodwork as blood urea nitrogen (BUN) in the US or urea nitrogen in other countries.

Not all amino acids can have the nitrogen removed outside of the body, so any normal keto acid analog is a mix of 5 keto acid analogs and 3 amino acids in all studies referenced in this book. You will see keto acid analogs referred to as KA in most cases, though sometimes it will be AA+KA, but they are the same thing.

Before going forward, let's put the amino acid question to bed first.

Let me address amino acid use as this is also a common question. Patients ask if they should take essential amino acids (EAA) instead of keto acid analogs (KA) when they reduce the protein in their diet. Amino acid supplementation had not been recommended in decades for kidney patients. When it was recommended, it was still noted that keto acid analogs were superior. We could not find a single study on amino acid supplementation for kidney patients in the last 30 years. We had to go all the way back to 1987–1994 to find studies. Several studies that we could find are listed below.

First study comparing KA vs amino acids

A crossover comparison of progression of chronic renal failure: Ketoacids (KA) versus amino acids (AA) (1993)[39]

Walser M, Hill SB, Ward L, Madger L (4 authors)

Number of Patients: 21 with CKD (but 5 dropped out)

Abstract: "For each patient, mean progression on KA was compared with mean progression on AA. Thirteen of 16 patients progressed slower on KA than AA. On the average, progression on KA was significantly slower (95% confidence limits GFR change = -0.36 to 0.09 ml/mm/month) than on AA (-0.91 to -0.41 ml/mm/month; $p = 0.024$). We conclude that KA slow progression, relative to AA, independently of protein or phosphorus intake, in patients on this regimen."

Easy-to-Read Summary: Researchers designed a head-to-head comparison of keto acid analogs and amino acids. Patients did not know what they were getting, and the researchers switched them every few months. People taking the keto acid analogs had much better GFRs compared to those that took amino acids.

Second study showing benefit of KA over amino acids

Progression of chronic renal failure on substituting a keto acid supplement for an amino acid supplement (1992)[40]

Walser M, Hill S, Ward L (3 authors)

Number of Patients: 12 with CKD

Abstract: "[Patients received] an essential amino acid supplement and were then switched to a keto acid supplement, while continuously receiving a very low-protein (0.3 g/kg), low-phosphorus (7 to 9 mg/kg) diet. Urinary urea excretion indicated that actual dietary protein intake averaged 0.46 g/kg. The results suggest that this keto acid supplement slows progression by approximately half, compared with an essential amino acid supplement, with no change in diet."

Easy-to-Read Summary: Researchers gave one group of people with CKD a regular essential amino acid supplement. They gave a second group of people with CKD a keto acid supplement. Both groups had low protein diets. The people who took the keto acid supplement had much better kidney function (twice as good) compared to the other group.

Third study comparing effects of KA versus amino acids

Adaptive responses to very low protein diets: The first comparison of ketoacids to essential amino acids (1994)[41]

Masud T, Young VR, Chapman T, Maroni BJ (4 authors)

Number of Patients: 8 with CKD over 15 days with lots of special testing

Conclusion: "Finally, evidence indicating that a VLPD supplemented with KA slows progression compared to an identical diet plus EAA [essential amino acids] while maintaining neutral BN [nitrogen balance] despite a lower nitrogen content, suggests a therapeutic advantage for KA over EAA."

Easy-to-Read Summary: Researchers found volunteers with CKD and had them stay in the hospital for a few weeks so they could control their diet. One group had a VLPD with essential amino acid supplement; the other group had a VLPD with ketoacid supplement. The keto acid analog group slowed disease progression compared to amino acids.

Fourth study comparing KA and amino acids

Progression of chronic renal failure in patients given keto acids following amino acids (1987)[42]

Walser M, LaFrance ND, Ward L, Van Duyn MA (4 authors)

Number of Patients: 12 CKD patients who were getting sicker on a VLPD with essential amino acid supplements.

Abstract: "Thus, this keto acid supplemented regimen apparently halted the progression of moderately-severe chronic renal failure [CKD] for at least a year in a small group of patients in whom restriction of protein and phosphate intake without keto acids failed to halt progression. In more severe renal failure, no effect on progression was seen."

Easy-to-Read Summary: *Of the initial 12 patients, half were switched from an essential amino acid supplement to a keto acid supplement, and all of them who stayed on the VLPD+KA avoided dialysis—their kidney function stayed about the same over 1–2 years. Patients who were getting worse taking amino acids improved when they switched to keto acid analogs.*

Keto acid analogs are superior to amino acids in every study.

In head-to-head studies which really help us directly compare the 2 options, keto acid analogs were superior to regular amino acids in slowing kidney disease progression 100% of the time. No studies contradicted this finding and this is not new information. Dr. Mackenzie Walser from Johns Hopkins University also published similar guidance 20 years ago in the 2004 edition of *Coping with Kidney Disease*.[43] The reason there have been no new studies about this is because the question was answered some time ago. Disease progression was slowed by as much as 50% in one study when the only change was from amino acids to keto acid analogs.

Amino acids do not lower the nitrogen load enough to benefit us or do not provide other benefits associated with keto acid analogs. Essential amino acids have from 1,200–1,600 mg of nitrogen per day that the kidneys have to work to eliminate. This is only a very slight reduction in nitrogen load when compared to normal dietary intake of nitrogen, so no benefit could be found.

The keto acid analogs used in the studies contained up to 864 mg of supplemental nitrogen or almost 50% less than amino acids. It's very clear that every milligram of nitrogen matters when your kidneys are not operating at 100%. More modern keto acid analogs have lowered the nitrogen load to less than 200 mg per day using a newer, patented technology leading to better outcomes. The lesson for patients is that every aspect of our dietary intake, including nitrogen content of protein supplements, will have an effect on our outcomes.

We had considered this a settled issue. However, the 2024 KDIGO[2] surprised us by recommending both amino acids and keto acid analogs without differentiation. The implication is amino acids and keto acid analogs are equal in outcomes. No study of amino acids is referenced in the 2024 KDIGO, so we can't find any studies or document any evidence used to make this recommendation.[2] We assume this recommendation is due to lack of keto acid analog availability in some countries. The 2020 KDOQI[1] does not recommend amino acid supplementation, so we have conflicting recommendations here. However, the 2020 KDOQI and 2024 KDIGO both recommend keto acid analogs.

Supplementing amino acids using pills or protein powders is normally a very bad practice for us as you can see. These pills or powders are simply concentrated forms of amino acids.

All available evidence is that kidney disease progresses faster if you are taking amino acids when compared to keto acid analogs. No published evidence exists to the contrary.

Back to keto acid analogs and establishing a benefit or not

We know keto acid analogs are better for us than amino acid supplements. But, let's try to answer another question: can keto acid analogs improve outcomes on LPD? This is an interesting question as LPD should not need protein supplementation. RDAs are being met, or close to being met, by dietary intake alone on traditional LPD. Keto acid analogs should only prove beneficial if something other than protein nutrition is involved or maybe if protein nutrition on LPD was inadequate.

We know that changing from amino acids to keto acid analogs slowed kidney disease progression by up to 50% and in a clinically significant way from the studies above. However, what will happen when people add a keto acid analog to low protein diets (LPD) when keto acid analogs are not really needed?

One meta-analysis will be combined with individual studies to answer this question.

First study on importance of KA for those with CKD

The effect of keto-analogues on chronic kidney disease deterioration: A meta-analysis (2019)[44]

Li A, Lee HY, Lin YC (3 authors)

Number of Patients: 951 from 10 randomized control trials (RCTs) and 2 non-RCTs

Abstract: "The protein-restricted KA-treated patients in this large series showed no statistically significant change during the 1-year study period, indicating slowing down of progression of CKD. In addition, there was an improvement in metabolic status and nutrition, although the protein-restricted diet in normal circumstances is likely to cause malnutrition...."

"A restricted protein diet supplemented with ketoanalogues (KA) was found to significantly delay the progression of CKD particularly in patients with an estimated glomerular filtration rate (eGFR) > 18 mL/min/1.73 m^2. No significant change in eGFR was found when comparing a very-low-protein diet and a low-protein diet. In conclusion, KA could slow down the progression of CKD in patients with eGFR > 18 mL/min/1.73 m2 without causing malnutrition and reverse CKD-MBD [chronic kidney disease with mineral and bone disorder] in patients with eGFR < 18 mL/min/1.73 m^2."

Easy-to-Read Summary*: This meta-analysis looked at many studies with LPDs and VLPDs, with and without KAs. They found that adding KA to a restricted protein diet helped slow kidney disease and reversed mineral and bone disorder. Kidney disease showed no real progression over a 1-year period in patients taking KA, which is noteworthy.*

Second study showing benefit of KA

The role of a low protein diet supplemented with ketoanalogues on kidney progression in pre-dialysis chronic kidney disease patients (2023)[45]

Ariyanopparut S, Kamonchanok M, Avihingsanon Y, Ong SE, Kittiskulnam P (5 authors)

Number of Patients: 1,042 patients with CKD on LPD (about half also took KA for at least 6 months)

Abstract: "During a median follow-up of 32.9 months, patients treated with LPD–KAs had a significantly lower risk of kidney function decline and dialysis initiation than LPD alone after adjusting for confounders. The annual rate of eGFR decline in patients receiving LPD–KAs was 4.5 mL/min/1.73 m^2 compared with 7.7 mL/min/1.73 m^2 in LPD alone. According to KAs dose–response analysis, the daily dose of ≤ 5 tablets was conversely associated with a higher risk of the primary endpoint, whereas the association disappeared among patients receiving a dose of > 6 tablets.[4]"

Easy-to-Read Summary*: The CKD patients who followed an LPD alone (without KA) were more likely to start dialysis, and their eGFR fell by -7.7 mL/min/1.73 m^2 each year on average. The CKD patients who followed LPD and used KA had their eGFR fall by about only -4.5 mL/min/1.73 m^2 or half as many points per year on average. They also looked at how many KA tablets were needed to get the most benefit and found it was 5–6. (This translates to 3.5 g per day of keto acid analogs or 4 Albutrix pills).*

---

4   Six tablets in this study is the same as 3.5 g of KA, which can be found in 4 Albutrix pills.

The numbers reported in this study about GFR decline confirm our finding of almost identical rates of GFR decline on LPD and VLPD+KA diets.

Third study showing positive effects of KA

Effect of essential amino acid ketoanalogues and protein restriction diet on morphogenetic proteins (FGF-23 and klotho) in 3B-4 stages chronic kidney disease patients: A randomized pilot study (2018)[46]

Milovanova L, Fomin V, Moiseev S, et al (11 authors)

Number of Patients: 79 patients with CKD 3B–4 and without diabetes on LPD (half also got KA supplements)

Conclusion: "LPD + KA provides support for nutrition status and contributes to more efficient correction of FGF-23 and Klotho abnormalities that may result in cardiovascular calcification and cardiac remodeling decreasing in CKD. At the same time, a prolonged LPD alone may lead to malnutrition."

Easy-to-Read Summary: *Adding KA to an LPD can help prevent malnutrition and help prevent heart disease signs.*

Fourth study showing positive effects of KA for CKD patients

Effect of low protein diet supplemented with ketoanalogues on endothelial function and protein-bound uremic toxins in patients with chronic kidney disease (2023)[47]

Chang G, Shih HM, Pan CF, Wu CJ, Lin CJ (5 authors)

Number of Patients: 22 CKD 3B–4 patients on LPD, half also got KA

Abstract: "LPD supplemented with KAs significantly preserves kidney function and provides additional benefits on endothelial function and protein-bound uremic toxins in patients with CKD."

Easy-to-Read Summary: *CKD patients who followed an LPD and also took KA supplements had better kidney function, better blood flow, and fewer hard-to-remove toxins than patients who followed an LPD alone.*

Fifth study of KA's positive effects on disease progression

Influence of ketoanalogues supplementation on the progression in chronic kidney disease patients who had training on low-protein diet (2009)[48]

Chang JH, Kim DK, Park JT, et al (10 authors)

Number of Patients: 120 participants with CKD 3–4. First, patients were started on LPD alone for 6 months, then LPD + KA for 6 months.

Results: "The declining slopes of glomerular filtration rate (GFR) during the LPD + KA period were significantly lower than those during the LPD alone period. This improvement in GFR was apparent in diabetic and non-diabetic subjects. However, serum albumin levels did not change… Responsiveness to LPD + KA was independently related to diabetes ($p = 0.006$) and high serum albumin levels ($p = 0.011$) in the LPD alone period."

Conclusion: "KA supplementation on over LPD delayed the progression of CKD without deteriorating nutritional status, and initial serum albumin levels could be an independent factor."

Easy-to-Read Summary: *When patients who were already on LPD added KA, their GFR slopes improved. This was true whether or not they had diabetes.*

New and maybe groundbreaking information for us to consider

First, these studies are from the last 5 years, so this is new information for almost everyone. The results of 2,200 patients and 30 physicians/researchers may change how we manage kidney disease in the future.

Second, it's groundbreaking information because 100% of these studies go against traditional guidance for LPD by supplementing protein with keto acid analogs. Increasing protein intake with keto acid analogs should have worsened results using traditional logic for kidney diets, but that is the opposite of what happened.

Instead, every study without exception documented that keto acid analogs improved outcomes for people on LPD by slowing kidney disease progression. No conflicting data exists on this subject. The clear implication is that keto acid analogs are the reason patients improved, not the dietary approach (LPD). Rates of progression are almost identical for LPD+KA and VLPD+KA in these studies. This is a surprising finding and raises the question: what is going on? What aspects of keto acid analogs are providing the benefits?

Thankfully, no one is dissecting humans, so we had to look for animal studies.[49]

Keto acid analogs protected mice from metabolic disorders, reduced inflammation, and **slowed the rate of fibrosis or scarring** in multiple studies. This is very interesting as we are trying to slow the rates of scarring or fibrosis and correct metabolic problems to improve our kidney function.

This study on mice demonstrated that keto acid analogs achieved the following benefits:

- Lower creatinine levels
- Lower BUN levels

- Lowered renal damage

- Lowered proinflammatory cytokine levels (a marker for inflammation)

- Lowered malondialdehyde levels (a marker for inflammation)

The benefits of keto acid analogs when used with LPD in humans were likely related to corrected metabolic dysfunction, reduced oxidative stress, reduced inflammation, lower rates of scarring/fibrosis and improved levels of hormones that normally decline with declining kidney function, too. We would like evidence that some or all of these benefits occurred in humans and not just mice. Evidence from animal studies is helpful, but I am always uncomfortable with the more subjective evidence or not understanding the underlying mechanism for improvement. Time to dig a little deeper.

Next study showing KA's value in advanced CKD

Ketoanalogue supplements (KA) reduce mortality in patients with pre-dialysis advanced diabetic kidney disease: A nationwide population-based study (2021)[50]

Chen HY, Sun CY, Lee CC, et al (8 authors)

Number of Patients: 15,782 patients with Stage 5 CKD caused by diabetes who haven't started dialysis. About 6% of them used KA.

Discussion: "We found that the KA users had a significantly lower risk of death during the follow-up period, and notably, the survival benefit of KAs increased in parallel with increasing cumulative dose and duration. We also found that the KA users were significantly associated with lower risks of developing coronary artery disease, cerebrovascular accidents, and major adverse cardiovascular events."

Easy-to-Read Summary: These researchers followed over 15,000 patients with CKD 5 to see if KA was helpful. People who used KAs lived longer on average than people who didn't. The people who used KA also had fewer heart attacks, heart diseases, and strokes. The people who used more KAs and who used them longer had better results than the people who used less KA supplementation.

Next study showing positive effects of KA on muscle mass

Effects of ketoanalogues on skeletal muscle mass in patients with advanced chronic kidney disease: Real-world evidence (2021)[51]

Lin YL, Hou JS, Wang CH, Su CY, Lio HH, Hsu BG (6 authors)

Number of Patients: 148 CKD patients. Some used KA, some didn't. Their muscle mass was measured over time.

Results: "KA users tended to maintain skeletal muscle and body fat mass, whereas non-KA users had a significantly reduced muscle mass ($p = 0.011$) and body fat gain ($p = 0.004$). Stratified by median age, in patients ≥68 y of age, non-KA users yielded the most significant muscle mass reduction and fat mass gain, whereas KA users revealed no changes in skeletal muscle and fat mass."

Conclusion: "In real-world practice, we concluded that KA supplementation favorably prevents skeletal muscle mass loss and fat mass gain in elderly patients with stage 4–5 CKD."

Easy-to-Read Summary: *Researchers looked at CKD patients who took KA and CKD patients who didn't take KA and measured their muscles and fat over time. People who took KA kept their muscles and didn't gain body fat. People who didn't use KA gained body fat and lost muscle. This was seen in every age group, but the most dramatic gains in body fat and muscle loss were in people aged 68 or older.*

A lot of new information for us to consider

Now, we have more data covering 18,000 patients, 63 physicians, and over 20 studies with head-to-head comparisons present very compelling and high quality evidence.

Evidence based on GFR/eGFR and BUN levels:

1. 100% of studies on keto acid analogs documented a benefit in slowing rates of kidney disease progression. Keto acid analogs added to LPD slowed progression from -7.5% to -4.5% when keto acid analogs were the only change. GFR trajectories are now almost identical on LPD+KA and VLPD+KA. The idea or concept that diet is less important than keto acid analog use is a new concept and goes against previous guidance or expectations.

2. BUN levels did not reach normal ranges in studies that reported BUN levels which is a negative.

Other relevant data:

1. A lower risk of death and lower rates of heart disease reported in stage 5 patients is very surprising and noteworthy. This large study again implies that the benefits of KA extend well beyond traditional protein nutrition.

2. Losing muscle mass is a common concern for patients on low or very low protein diets, but keto acid analogs appear to allow for better retention of muscle mass.

3. In the past, it was thought that LPD did not need protein supplementation with keto acid analogs, but this appears to be 100% incorrect based on new data. LPD supplemented with keto acid analogs appear to provide better nutrition or other

benefits that lead to improved albumin levels and better GFR trajectories. LPD may be deficient in ways we don't understand otherwise adding keto acid analogs would not have improved outcomes to this extent.

4. A dose-response relationship exists, and a minimum effective dose or serving of keto acid analogs further documents that benefits are from keto acid analogs and not another dietary source.

5. Animal studies and human studies both document slower fibrosis or scarring of kidneys when keto acid analogs are used. Keto acid analogs acted as a protective factor in 100% animal studies we found. The implication is that keto acid analogs are solving more problems than they create. On the other hand, amino acids may be contributing to more problems than they solve.

Some negatives to consider for LPD+KA

Two clear negatives are that GFR decline is still within the normal rates of progression (-4.5%) and BUN levels were not returned to normal in any study that reported BUN. We did not find any data on higher protein diets (greater than 0.8 g/kg/day) with keto acid analogs, so if there is a benefit, it is unknown for diets higher in protein.

We still did not get what we are after, but adding keto acid analogs to LPD or a less restrictive diet may represent an option for patients who are not willing to go on lower protein diets and are willing to accept a somewhat slower decline as the outcome.

If someone or a company is recommending amino acids or keto acid analogs or any other form of protein supplementation, please go over this chapter with them to decide what is best for you.

For patients, I wanted to list some key points that are essential to our education on kidney disease diets.

You should know

1. Protein restriction **alone** has no published record of success in slowing kidney disease progression to rates slower than normal disease progression or achieving normal BUN levels. This is true for both low protein (LPD) and very low protein diets (VLPD).

2. Keto acid analogs **alone** have no published record of success in slowing kidney disease progression to rates slower than normal disease progression or achieving normal BUN levels.

3. Plant-based diets **alone** have no published record of success in slowing kidney disease progression or achieving normal BUN levels.

4. Amino acids **alone** or **combined** with diets have no published record of success in slowing kidney disease progression with or without different diets.

5. **Only** authentic or real keto acid analogs like those used in studies have a record of any improvements(Albutrix S3,S4,S5 or Ketosteril). Hybrid amino acid/keto acid analog products or amino acids have no published record of success.

6. **No** past published combination of diets, keto acid analogs, or amino acids achieved our goals of slowing kidney disease to rates slower than normal disease progression or achieving normal BUN levels.

Maybe things are not as confusing as we thought. Most issues are very, very clear with minimal conflicting data when we equally apply the same objective standards.

I will also keep saying this for emphasis—*this is the real reason why these diets or dietary combinations are not mainstream medicine today.* Clinically significant outcomes could not be documented compared to normal disease progression rates.

Patient self defense

This section has enough data for you to use to check any recommendations made to you by physicians, dieticians, nutritionists, friends, websites, diet books, or anywhere else. I hope this section will dramatically reduce confusion regarding kidney diets and expected outcomes for different dietary combinations.

You can also clearly see that the general recommendations we get like reducing protein, eating healthier, trying a mediterranean diet, going plant based, etc.. have no proof of effectiveness on their own.

We also have some hard and fast limitations going forward. We know .6 g/kg of protein is too much whether the protein or diet is plant or animal. We also know that anything below .3 g/kg is unsustainable or unachievable in real life in terms of protein restriction. We also know that keto acid analogs should be used instead of amino acids.

As you can clearly see, the lack of a regulatory standard or objective standards is an absolute killer for us if we are not educated.

Now, let's dive into emerging evidence, newer technologies, theories and a possible breakthrough on how we can actually slow kidney disease progression consistently and by very meaningful amounts.

Part 3: Going into Theory and Emerging Evidence

As stated, I organized this book into parts, because we went from largely proven issues with a large amount of research in Part 2 to new evidence and theories in Part 3. I wanted to go to great pains to point out these differences.

At Kidneyhood.org, we have a definite theory on how to manage kidney disease so as to preserve your kidneys and lose as few nephrons as possible over the coming years. This theory is backed by my experience as a 25+year kidney patient, 2 small studies to date and anecdotal data from hundreds of patients. Few things replace decades of being a kidney patient trying to improve or change your outcome, yet my personal experience is worthless from a statistical perspective (1 patient vs many), despite being what's guided us from the start. So, like any good researcher, I want to be clear that these results are still early. That's why our results are separate from the other research in the book. We will be covering theories about kidney disease progression and new patented technologies in this section.

As patients, ideally, we need a method to slow kidney disease progression to a rate slower than normal kidney disease progression. We need to improve measurably so that we know for sure that diet or dietary combination is impacting our future outcome. For clinicians, we need to prove our program with a clinical standard in several trials or studies before they will begin to accept or recommend any dietary approach to kidney disease. We need to eliminate subjectiveness or subjective claims when we can.

We need to be able to prove effectiveness to a standard that resembles a clinical standard used to approve drugs before mainstream adoption can take place. After all, if we cannot prove effectiveness, then we will still be stuck in the current chaos with too many unknowns.

I hope our observations and research will help you greatly in the future. For the most updated information, please see our website at www.kidneyhood.org or email us at support@kidneyhood.org.

Chapter 9

The Dysfunctions and Damage Approach to Kidney Disease Management

I want to give you another way to think about managing kidney disease. I believe the concepts in this chapter should be the bedrock or base for any successful approach to kidney disease management. I want you to think about your overall health and recent blood tests now and forget about diets for a few chapters.

Section 1: Dysfunctions

Dysfunctions drive kidney disease progression

For our purposes here, we will consider any measurement, blood test, or urine test outside the normal or healthy range to be a *dysfunction*. A *dysfunction* could be high blood pressure or high BUN levels, body weight well above a healthy weight, phosphorus outside the normal range, Type 2 diabetes, and so on. A dysfunction is something not working properly or outside the normal range , so we have to compensate for this issue or take steps to correct it.

The more dysfunctions you have or the more severe those dysfunctions are, the worse the trajectory of your GFR and your overall health will be. If we know this to be true, and it is, then solving, treating, or effectively managing dysfunctions should be the goal of any patient education program, kidney diets, keto acid analogs, vitamins, lifestyle changes, nutritional interventions, kidney-related books etc.

The only difference between you and a healthy patient is simply the number of dysfunctions you have. The healthy patient has no dysfunctions, but we as kidney patients normally have several common dysfunctions. If we can eliminate, solve, or treat every dysfunction, then our future outcomes should look more like a normal or healthy person in theory.

Our primary goal should be to solve every dysfunction.

Decreasing the number of dysfunctions is also the model for successful aging and heart disease management, so this model is a winner on several levels. If we solve every health issue as it pops up, our odds of living longer, higher-quality lives go up. If we let health problems or dysfunctions increase in severity or number, our life expectancy and quality of life will be lower.

Let me give you some examples of dysfunctions that can speed up kidney disease progression. It may help give you an idea of the complexity and the number of issues we need to manage successfully. Your dietary intake compared with your current kidney function can affect all of these issues, and this is just a partial list.

- Uremia (high BUN levels)
- Specific uremic toxins
- Inflammation
- Acidosis
- Low albumin levels
- Proteinuria (protein or albumin in your urine)
- Sodium outside the normal range
- Potassium outside the normal range
- Phosphorus outside the normal range
- Oxidative stress
- Unhealthy weight or body mass index (BMI)
- High calcium levels
- Low magnesium levels
- Blood pressure that is too high or too low
- Advanced glycation product levels (from smoking or burned parts of foods)
- High glycemic vs low glycemic diet consequences
- Effective diabetes (both Type 1 and Type 2) management
- Endothelial dysfunction (reduced blood flow, narrowing, or stiffening of arteries)
- Anemia

- Vitamin D deficiency

- And more[56-63]

We have to properly compensate for our reduced kidney function for every issue on this list (and more) if we can. Each dysfunction comes with its own specific strategies that may be used to bring it back to normal. The hard part is all of these strategies must be used simultaneously to solve as many dysfunctions as possible. The movie title *Everything, Everywhere, All at Once* is a good way to describe what we have to do on kidney diets. We have to address every dysfunction successfully at the same time. Solving one dysfunction while creating another dysfunction will not help us, and this happened frequently in past approaches to kidney disease management.

So, the real job of any kidney diet is to accurately compensate for our reduced kidney function so that we have no dysfunctions while achieving the RDAs for nutrition. Objective evidence of accurate compensation is normal or much improved blood and urine tests.

Every dysfunction drives a cascade of dysfunctions.

Dysfunctions don't exist in isolation. Every dysfunction has an associated cascade of dysfunctions that work to speed up kidney disease progression and degrade our overall health. Each known dysfunction contributes to multiple other health problems that are rarely measured. There are no exceptions to this rule.

Staying with the blood urea nitrogen or BUN example, we want our BUN levels to be normal for a reason. As our kidney disease progresses, our BUN levels start to rise because we cannot excrete these wastes faster than they are building up in our bloodstream. The microscopic scarred filters in our kidneys are unable to keep up with the workload. We start a cascading effect of bad things leading to more bad things. Many related dysfunctions also work to increase the speed of kidney disease progression.

On your blood test, imagine only BUN is higher than the normal range. This contributes to the following cascades of dysfunctions:

- Decreased beneficial bacteria in gut microbiome

- Overgrowth of other bacteria leading to imbalance

- Because of microbiome issues, impaired protein/amino acid metabolism

- Protein-energy wasting or malnutrition

- Increased/accelerated cardiovascular disease

- Faster kidney disease progression
- Insulin resistance/less insulin secretion
- Immune system issues (increased antibiotic use)
- Slower wound healing[60]
- Increased inflammation
- Increased oxidative stress
- Higher chance of getting anemia[13]
- High rate of hospitalization
- Increased odds of dialysis
- Higher mortality (death) rates[65]
- And more.[66,67]

One dysfunction (high BUN levels) leads to dozens of potential dysfunctions, which can be known or unknown, measured or unmeasured.

The lesson is that any dysfunction we leave untreated or unmanaged spawns a long list of other problems that contribute to kidney and heart disease progression. There are no exceptions to this rule. Every dysfunction has a related cascade of dysfunctions degrading our health and making it harder to slow kidney disease progression.

A few more examples will drive this point home.

High sodium levels contribute to

- Faster kidney disease progression
- High blood pressure (hypertension)
- Heart failure
- Enlarged heart muscle (unhealthy and weaker)
- Edema or swelling[68]
- Kidney stones[69]
- Lower calcium absorption/osteoporosis[70]
- Stomach cancer[71]

- Stroke

- Increased mortality (death) rates[68]

Bringing your sodium levels back to the normal range solves or reduces the risks of a lot of dysfunctions, some of which you may never have associated with salt intake—like stomach cancer or kidney stones. Recently, a study showed limiting sodium to 1,500 mg per day was as effective as a drug for reducing blood pressure.[72] Correcting or managing dietary issues can be very powerful—far more effective than most people think.

Phosphorus is another example of a common issue for kidney patients. The normal range for serum phosphorus is 3.4–4.5 mg/dL (1.12–1.45 mmol/L).

Phosphorus dysfunctions are associated with the following cascade of dysfunctions:

- Worsened heart disease

- Increased rates of vascular calcifications (the number one killer of kidney patients)

- Increased oxidative stress

- Increased endothelial dysfunction (hardening or narrowing of arteries)

- Increased rate of kidney disease progression[73]

- Increased inflammation, worsening anemia and muscle wasting.[74]

To be even more clear: **every 1 mg/dL increase in phosphorus was independently associated with an increased rate of kidney failure.**[73]

Once again, the lesson is that every dysfunction has a related cascade of health problems created by a dysfunction. <u>These related dysfunctions are rarely measured, tested, or managed and that is a big problem for us.</u> Protein restriction helps with some issues, but not enough to actually change our future outcome. Protein restriction may be needed, but we can't ignore the dozens of other dysfunctions that may speed up kidney disease progression.

Every dysfunction independently drives kidney disease progression.

<u>A further complication to our situation is the fact that every dysfunction affects our future outcome *independent* of other dysfunctions. Understanding this fact should be a cornerstone of all kidney education.</u>

Let's assume we have everything in the normal range with only one dysfunction, like the BUN example. High BUN levels, or uremia, harm our kidneys and increase the speed of kidney disease progression even if everything else is perfect. The same is true for things like phosphorus, sodium, oxidative stress, inflammation, blood pressure, diabetes etc.

Because these dysfunctions work independently to damage our kidneys even when everything else is perfect, this evidence means every dysfunction must be solved or managed at the same time and for a long period of time if we really want to improve our overall health and try to slow disease progression.

The proper way manage kidney disease for life

Our current theory is that successful kidney disease management is based on the number and severity of dysfunctions solved more than any other factor.

Let me repeat this again for emphasis:

Slowing kidney disease progression or successful kidney disease management is primarily based on the number and or severity of dysfunctions solved more than any other factor.

We see overwhelmingly the patients who improve GFR the most are the ones solving the most dysfunctions. We see it day after day. The patients taking the time and making the effort to improve their overall health are the ones with the biggest improvements in kidney-related measures and quality of life.

As an example, patients who enter a kidney diet study with 3 dysfunctions and keep those same dysfunctions through the study, do not improve on average or only slightly improve. The patients that do improve are the ones lowering the number and severity of dysfunctions.

If you never take steps to get healthier overall, your odds of success are slim to none. It's a pure myth or mirage that you can let your overall health degrade or worsen and still slow kidney disease progression.

The most successful study from the previous section was a VLPD+KA plant-based diet with the author stating the following:

"The favorable effects of the...[very low protein plant-based diet with keto acid analogs] seem to be mediated more by the correction of metabolic complications of advanced CKD, notably the improvement in nitrogen balance, mineral metabolism disturbances, metabolic acidosis, and inflammation, than by reduction in GFR decline."[28]

The same concept was noted in LPD+KA vs LPD studies. Authentic keto acid analogs improved metabolic and nutritional status, improved hormone levels, reduced uremic toxins, etc. which together slowed rates of kidney disease progression compared to LPD alone.

We see a difference in the outcome on LPD vs VLPD+KA in speeds of kidney disease progression, but we also see a reduction in the severity of BUN levels with VLPD+KA. The dysfunction of high BUN levels was partially solved using VLPD+KA, but not on LPD.

The implication here is that correcting dysfunctions—like mineral disturbances, inflammation, acidosis, oxidative stress and dozens of related cascades is the way we improve our odds with kidney disease. Solving multiple dysfunctions can lead to very dramatic improvements as the patient's health changes dramatically.

A dysfunctions approach to kidney disease management also explains past failures

What we like about this approach is we can see more clearly or explain why previous approaches may not have worked or been effective.

Low protein diets(LPD) did not improve blood and urine tests on average, so no dysfunctions were solved.

Low protein diets + keto acid analogs (LPD+KA) solved or improved some dysfunctions like improving metabolic status/nutrition, reversing mineral-bone disorders, reduced uremic toxins etc.. so some dysfunctions were solved or reduced, but others were allowed to worsen(like BUN). For these reasons, some improvements were documented.

Very low protein diets (VLPD+KA) solved some dysfunctions by lowering BUN levels by - 20%, so some improvements were documented.

Plant based diets did not improve blood and urine tests on average, so no dysfunctions were solved. We see evidence of this fact with every variation of traditional diets.

Amino acids did not improve blood and urine tests on average, so no dysfunctions were solved. No benefit was documented.

Keto acid analogs likely improved metabolic issues, slowed fibrosis or scarring and reduced oxidative stress and inflammation. BUN levels are also improved. Several dysfunctions were likely solved or reduced in number, so a measurable benefit was documented.

The clear message is any improvements from a dietary approach are directly related to reducing the severity and number of dysfunctions more than any other factor. A dysfunctional view of kidney disease can now drive our approach to kidney disease management which should lead to greatly improved outcomes.

Section 2: Managing Dysfunctions Successfully

Going after the root cause is the proper way to solve dysfunctions.

Staying with the dysfunctions model, we need to decide how to deal with both known and unknown dysfunctions.

We must treat, solve, correct, or manage dysfunctions at their root cause. This is the only strategy that works effectively to address dysfunctions and improve our overall health. Let me explain this very important issue in detail.

We often confuse symptoms with dysfunctions, but they are different. Treating or managing symptoms does not improve our health in most cases. Solving the problem at the root cause is the only approach to eliminate dysfunctions that also reduces the number and severity of related cascades of dysfunctions. The evidence proves that if we never solve the underlying health problems and just manage symptoms, our disease still progresses.

Let me give you a few examples to make sure you understand this important point.

Normal ranges can be ghostbusters.

A good example of *ghostbusting* is uremic itching, also called uremic pruritus or chronic kidney disease-associated pruritus. The exact cause of uremic itching is a bit like a ghost that is hard to pin down. There are many theories, but no one knows the exact cause. High blood urea nitrogen, high phosphorus and high calcium levels have all been labeled as possible causes.[75] The effect is patients develop itchy skin with differing intensities. Some patients tell us it is literally driving them crazy. Historically, treatment options are creams, antihistamines, or steroids for the symptoms, but these do not solve the root cause.[76]

We refer to conditions with no established cause as *ghosts*. We have found that bringing blood tests back into the normal ranges are *ghostbusters* in many cases. Bringing all blood tests back into the normal ranges appears to slow and then stop uremic itching in all cases to date. In the past, a transplant was considered the only real cure for uremic itching. Of course, a transplant has the same effect of returning blood work to normal or solving the dysfunction. Same solution, but a very different approach.

Once the root dysfunction(s) of out-of-range blood tests are solved, itching starts to improve and then normally goes away completely. Accurate dietary compensation for diseased kidneys is likely much more effective than pills and creams for uremic itching.

We always get bonuses to our overall health when we solve the root dysfunction.

The bonus of solving the dysfunction of uremic itching at the root cause is that we likely solved a large number of related dysfunctions and related cascades by bringing all blood tests back to normal. We actually became measurably healthier using this approach. This doesn't happen with antihistamines, creams, or just managing symptoms.

Probiotics, unintended consequences, common sense and root causes

Probiotics are a good example of good intentions without addressing the root causes. Many patients report taking probiotics in an attempt to change something likely unmeasurable like *gut health*. We need to apply some *root cause* common sense to many issues.

High blood urea nitrogen (BUN) levels are known to impair or degrade at least some of the bacteria in our gut, which may cause impaired blood urea nitrogen metabolism, which, in turn, leads to even higher blood urea nitrogen levels through a dysregulated or impaired microbiome.[77] Probiotics use is a legitimate consideration.

However, we need some common sense to guide us here. If we think something in our gut microbiome is wrong, we need to ask " Why is it wrong?" Supplementing probiotics while BUN levels are high is somewhat useless exercise. We send the probiotics to their death or impairment because we never corrected the root cause of our suspected impaired microbiome. In addition, probiotic supplements are limited to the 15–20 strains that can be cost-effectively manufactured, not the 300+ strains in your gut. The end result is we never corrected the underlying issue (high BUN levels), and we supplemented 1% -1.5% of all the strains in our gut. We left the other 98.5%–99% of strains to be impaired. Lastly, no measurement tool exists, so it's completely subjective when you try to evaluate results. We never know if something is working or not in this case.

If we don't treat the root causes and only treat the symptoms, we may also end up with unintended consequences. We are seeing this at an increasing rate as we work with more patients and gather more evidence. The evidence is building that supplements even as benign as probiotics may also change our future outcome.

The excerpt below is from an article summarizing a study that was validated in mice and then humans.[78] This study was on cancer patients taking probiotics vs a high-fiber diet, but it serves as a good example about root causes, shortcuts, and unintended consequences. I found this while researching options for my sister who was fighting a very aggressive form of cancer at the time, but it made an impression on me in terms of symptoms vs dysfunctions.

"People who reported higher fiber intake, which promotes healthy gut microbes, had better responses to treatment overall. After adjusting for other factors, the researchers found that every 5-gram increase in daily fiber intake corresponded to a 30% lower risk of cancer progression or death. Overall, people who ate the most fiber and didn't use probiotics had the best responses to immunotherapy. Probiotics didn't appear to improve survival. In fact, the data suggested they might lower survival.

"In melanoma patients, taking over-the-counter probiotic supplements was associated with a 70 percent lower chance of response to cancer immunotherapy treatment."

Using our theory and the example above, we can clearly see that fiber intake likely solved more dysfunctions than probiotic intake by addressing the root causes. 100% of our gut microbiome benefits from fiber intake compared with 1-1.5% possibly benefiting from probiotics. The finding that cancer patients may do worse with probiotic use is likely because no dysfunctions were ever treated, solved, or brought back to normal ranges by taking probiotics. Whatever dysfunctions existed before, still existed after taking probiotics.

My point here is not to advocate for or against probiotics, but to illustrate the proper way to think about solving or addressing dysfunctions. We never addressed the root cause, only supplemented 1% of gut bacteria and have no way to measure the effects.

Just like uremic itching, we get bonuses with fiber and reducing BUN levels

The bonus of a high-fiber diet and reducing BUN levels back to the normal ranges is that we are also solving dozens of related dysfunctions at the same time. We don't get this benefit if we just take probiotics while we let everything else worsen. We also solved uremic itching in most cases using the same approach.

Sodium bicarbonate

Another good example is sodium bicarbonate use in kidney patients. Sodium bicarbonate is very effective at reducing acid (metabolic acidosis) and considered very safe over the short term. It's one of the few supplements or medical foods with good data behind it.[79] However, sodium bicarbonate use has always been somewhat controversial as it is a form of sodium, and sodium is limited on kidney diets in most cases. Increased sodium intake increases blood pressure, so much so that recommended sodium intake for everyone may drop from 2,000 mg a day to around 1,500 mg a day based on new research that shows reducing sodium intake to 1,500 mg a day was as effective as a drug in lowering blood pressure.[72] One teaspoon of sodium bicarbonate contains 1,260 mg of sodium.[80]

If we are already consuming 2,000 mg of sodium per day from diet and every teaspoon of sodium bicarbonate adds 1,260 mg of sodium, then in every case, we are going well over the recommended limits for sodium intake. Many patients are consuming 5,000+ mg of sodium per day when everything is totaled and taking blood pressure medications at the same time. We are cranking up blood pressure with more salt intake, but then trying to crank it down with blood pressure drugs.

Increasing protein intake also requires greater amounts of sodium bicarbonate to correct the high dietary acid load, which in turn will normally require a higher dose of blood pressure medications.[81] It's a vicious circle, but it's one that is easy to stop.

While sodium bicarbonate is effective at treating the symptom (acidosis) and correcting acid levels, we never addressed the root cause of acidosis or the potentially dozens of other things wrong. The cause of acidosis is usually eating a diet that is too high in acid compared to your kidney's ability to correct the high acid levels. High BUN levels are also normally associated with acidosis. An alkaline or lower acid diet solves this problem at the root cause by reducing high-acid food intake to a level your current kidney function can handle. Acidosis normally becomes a thing of the past when you treat the root cause, and you don't have to worry about increased sodium intake, possible long-term risks of sodium bicarbonate use, or getting it just right with constant blood tests and adjustments. Heartburn and acid reflux also improve when a low-acid or alkaline diet is used.

Both patients on an alkaline diet (fruit/veggies diet) and those taking sodium bicarbonate lowered acidosis-related issues, but only one group had a reduction in blood pressure. Dietary approaches to acidosis lowered blood pressure, but sodium bicarbonate did not. **High blood pressure is the second leading cause of kidney disease, so these kinds of issues matter greatly to us.**

The other issue to be aware of is both high and low serum bicarbonate levels hurt our future outcomes, thus the amount of sodium bicarbonate patients take requires constant testing to ensure you are not too high or too low. The recommended range for serum bicarbonate levels is 24–26 mmol/L, a very narrow range. High supplemental intake creates risks we may not be aware of. Just blindly taking sodium bicarbonate has never been recommended by any reputable health organization, so be careful.

One last comment is that 150+ different drugs are listed as having potential interactions with sodium bicarbonate.[82] I can't find any interactions from eating a healthier diet lower in acid. Our life is more complicated than we think when we don't solve the problem at the root cause as you will see.

Again, there are more benefits just like solving the other root causes.

A low acid or alkaline diet normally solves the issue of acidosis and normally eliminates the need for sodium bicarbonate while lowering blood pressure, a major driver of kidney disease progression.

When you solved your acidosis or dietary acid load, you also likely solved lots of other dysfunctions as well. In this example, bringing your blood work back to normal ranges and eating an alkaline, high-fiber diet solved uremic itching, improved gut health and also reduced or eliminated the need for sodium bicarbonate. In terms of pill burden, you may no longer need antihistamines, steroids, probiotics, or sodium bicarbonate every day.

My point is if we are really trying to get healthier and taking our health seriously, we have to reduce the number of dysfunctions by going after the root causes. Treating or managing root causes always seems to have a lot of bonuses, and many of those bonuses effectively treat several root causes at the same time, correcting many health issues at once.

Treating symptoms rarely addresses the cause of the dysfunction and allows these dysfunctions to continue. Treating symptoms rarely has any bonuses except relief from the symptom. You are not getting healthier or reducing the drivers of kidney disease progression by treating symptoms. Remember, each dysfunction works against us independently, so every dysfunction needs to be treated at the root cause.

A big lesson for us

We have to improve the trajectory of our overall health if we want to change the trajectory of kidney disease progression. We improve the trajectory of our overall health by reducing the severity and number of dysfunctions at the root cause. Your overall health matters in every disease, and kidney disease is no exception. Again, it's a myth or mirage to think you can let your overall health worsen and still slow kidney disease progression (or any progressive disease).

There are no shortcuts in our experience despite what you read on the internet. No shortcuts is the bad news, but the good news is you can learn how to manage kidney disease in a short period of time (90 days or less), and once you learn those skills, you have them for life. That should be great news for us.

Chapter 10

Root Causes, Polypharmacy, and Our Future Outcomes (Pills Versus Diet and Lifestyle)

The lesson of solving dysfunctions at the root cause is so important. I wanted to drive home the key lesson of dysfunctions and root causes from a different perspective in this chapter. I wanted to compare what happens to us if we don't work on solving dysfunctions at the root cause.

The idea that diet and lifestyle changes are too hard completely falls apart when we look at what happens in real life. Getting sicker, dying younger, growing frailer, losing quality of life, increasing the number of health conditions, greater risk of drug interactions and soaring medical bills are much harder and more complex to manage compared to learning to manage kidney disease with diet, nutrition, education and lifestyle.

The least complicated and cheapest option is to keep your existing kidneys working as long as possible. Compare dialysis or transplant to eating healthy and accurately compensating for your diseased kidneys; it's not even close in terms of complexity, risks and costs.

Getting sicker is clearly the hardest road of all, but we unknowingly chose this route because we didn't think about the other side of the coin. Yes, I know you don't want to change your diet, but I also know you don't want to get sicker either.

The opposite of solving problems at the root cause might be *polypharmacy.*

Polypharmacy is a fancy way of saying *taking many pills* or *pill burden.* A more exact definition is the simultaneous use of multiple drugs by a single patient, for one or more conditions. The more pills we take, the more complicated our lives become, the sicker we are, and the worse our outcomes are. We rely on pills to solve issues and address symptoms instead of solving the problem at the root cause. Dialysis and transplant patients have the highest pill burdens of any group of kidney patients, and advanced kidney disease patients take more pills than the general population.[83]

Before diving into this, let me say that I am all for modern drugs. This chapter is not meant to inhibit or reduce the use of needed prescription drugs. The goal of this chapter is to accurately compare solving a problem at the root cause from the previous chapter to taking more pills and letting these dysfunctions continue or worsen. One way you are getting healthier, and the other way you are getting sicker in most cases. Never change or stop taking prescription drugs without your doctor's approval but don't be afraid to ask your doctor if there isn't a possibility to reduce the number of meds you take.

Each decision has an impact on our future outcome. Remember everything has a related, cascading effect on your health. Our goal here is to educate you on different outcomes associated with different choices.

First study on the negative effects of taking many medications

Polypharmacy in patients with chronic kidney disease (2024)[84]

Oosting IJ, Colombijn JMT, Kaasenbrood L, et al (9 authors)

Number of Patients: 63 studies with 484,915 patients in total

Results: "In patients with CKD, polypharmacy was associated with a higher risk of all-cause mortality, kidney failure, faster eGFR decline, lower quality of life (QoL), and higher medication non-adherence, adverse drug reactions, and potentially inappropriate medications."

Easy-to-Read Summary: People with kidney disease who took more medications were more likely to die, experience kidney failure, and have a lower quality of life compared to people with kidney disease who took fewer medications. The people who had many medications were also more likely to have problems with their medications.

Second study demonstrating negatives of many medications for CKD patients

Prevalence of polypharmacy and associated adverse health outcomes in adult patients with chronic kidney disease: Protocol for a systematic review and meta-analysis (2021)[85]

Okpechi IG, Tinwala MM, Muneer S, et al (23 authors)
Number of Patients: Unknown. This study has not been finished yet.

Background: "Polypharmacy has also been directly associated with mortality. In a systematic review that investigated the association between polypharmacy and mortality, a significant association between polypharmacy and death was observed when polypharmacy was defined as a discrete variable."

Easy-to-Read Summary: *When the number of drugs used is the only thing that is different between 2 groups of people, mortality (death) rates increase with taking an increasing number of prescription drugs.*

Third study showing the more medications CKD patients take, the worse their results are

Evaluation of the adequacy of drug prescriptions in patients with chronic kidney disease: Results from the CKD-REIN cohort (2018)[86]

Laville SM, Metzger M, Stengel B, et al (13 authors)

Number of Patients: 3033 outpatients with CKD (eGFR 15–60 mL/min/1.73 m^2)

Results: "Half of the patients had been prescribed at least one inappropriate drug. …The percentage of inappropriate prescriptions varied from one GFR equation to another: 52% when using the CKD-EPI equation, 47% when using the de-indexed CKD-EPI equation and 41% with the CG equation. …The risk of having at least one inappropriate prescription increased with the number of drugs per patient"

Easy-to-Read Summary: *The more prescription medications you take, the greater chance that one or more of the drugs you are taking is unsafe for kidney patients, may cause a bad and unintended reaction, or could interact with other drugs.*

Fourth study demonstrating worse health when CKD patients take more meds

Polypharmacy, chronic kidney disease, and mortality among older adults: A prospective study of National Health And Nutrition Examination Survey, 1999-2018 (2023)[87]

Wang X, Yang C, Jiang J, Hu Y, Hao Y, Dong JY (6 authors)

Number of Patients: 13,513 adults from 1999 to 2018 until December 31, 2019

Results: "Participants with polypharmacy had a 27% and 39% higher risk of all-cause and CVD mortality… Polypharmacy was associated with elevated risks of all-cause and CVD mortality among the elderly CKD patients."

Easy-to-Read Summary: *The more prescription drugs we take, the higher chance we will die or have a heart attack or stroke.*

Fifth study showing the more meds for CKD patients, the worse the outcome

Evaluation of drug-related problems in chronic kidney disease patients (2022)[88]

Shouqair TM, Rabbani SA, Sridhar SB, Kurian MT (4 authors)

Number of Patients: 130 patients with CKD

Abstract: "Drug-drug interactions and adverse drug reactions in CKD patients may lower the quality of life, increase the length of hospital stay, and augment the risks of morbidity and mortality....The mean number of drugs prescribed was 11.1 ± 3.8 per patient. The prevalence of potential drug-drug interactions was found to be 89.2%."

Easy-to-Read Summary: As you increase the number of drugs taken, the risks of undesired, harmful reactions or drug interactions increase as well. Almost 90% (89.2%) of patients were taking drugs that may have interactions or safety concerns when taken together.

Sixth study showing more meds have a deleterious effect on CKD patients

Association of polypharmacy with kidney disease progression in adults with CKD (2021)[89]

Kimura H, Tanaka K, Saito H, et al (11 authors)

Number of Patients: 1117 participants (median age, 66 years; 56% male; median eGFR, 48 ml/min/1.73 m^2) not on dialysis

Conclusion: "The use of a high number of medications was associated with a high risk of kidney failure, cardiovascular events, and all-cause mortality in Japanese patients with nondialysis-dependent CKD under nephrology care.

Easy-to-Read Summary: Kidney and heart disease progress faster in people who are taking a higher number of medications.

I could go on and on as many studies exist on this topic, but you get the idea. We have to increase the number of pills we take as dysfunctions worsen or go unsolved and our life is more complicated. Of course, not every condition or issue can be solved by diet, lifestyle, and nutrition, and some prescription drugs are considered best practices like blood pressure medications. However, when we can solve a health problem by diet, exercise, and lifestyle changes, clearly that is the best option—least complicated and least expensive in the long run.

In light of all this evidence, it makes sense to ask your doctor on a yearly basis to review your meds to determine if all of them are necessary. Remember most physicians see 1000–2000 patients in their practices. If you ask, then your physician is encouraged to determine if any medications could be eliminated or decreased.

Comorbid condition studies also show the value in solving health problems at the root cause.

A second way to look at a dysfunctions approach is *comorbid* conditions or the number of related health problems we have related to kidney disease. For us, comorbid conditions can be defined as dysfunctions related to reduced kidney function or diseased kidneys. Polypharmacy and comorbid conditions are 2 sides of the same coin.

As the number of comorbid conditions or dysfunction increases, so does the rate of kidney disease progression. As we let ourselves get sicker, we speed up kidney disease progression.

First study showing the negativity effects of comorbidity

Comorbidity as a driver of adverse outcomes in people with chronic kidney disease (2015)[90]

Tonelli M, Wiebe N, Guthrie B, et al (13 authors)

Number of Patients: 530,771 patients

Abstract: "Concordant comorbidities were associated with excess risk of hospitalization, but so were discordant comorbidities and mental health conditions. Thus, discordant comorbidities and mental health conditions as well as concordant comorbidities are important independent drivers of the adverse outcomes associated with CKD."

Note: Concordant in this case means associated with kidney disease. Discordants are health conditions not normally associated with kidney disease. Both are dysfunctions, and both appear to increase the speed of kidney disease progression.

Easy-to-Read Summary*: All dysfunctions, even the ones not normally related to kidney disease, increased the speed of kidney progression.*

Second study demonstrating the negative effect of comorbidities for CKD patients

The number of comorbidities predicts renal outcomes in patients with Stage 3–5 chronic kidney disease (2018)[91]

Lee WC, Lee YT, Li LC, et al (9 authors)

Discussion: "More importantly, our data demonstrate a link between multimorbidity and worse renal outcomes. As multi comorbidity has been shown to increase both disease and treatment burden in CKD patients…"

Easy-to-Read Summary: *The more dysfunctions or comorbid conditions you have, the faster kidney disease progresses.*

Third study showing negative aspects of comorbidity for CKD patients

Comorbidity in chronic kidney disease: A large cross-sectional study of prevalence in Scottish primary care (2021)[92]

MacRae C, Mercer SW, Guthrie B, Henderson D (4 authors)

Number of Patients: Analysis of data of 1,274,374 adults in Scotland (33,567 with CKD)

Results: "Furthermore, all concordant (seven out of seven), the majority of discordant physical health conditions (17 out of 24), and mental health conditions (six out of eight) had statistically significant positive associations with CKD after adjustment."

Easy-to-Read Summary: Again, every health condition contributes to the speed of kidney disease progression, even when these conditions are not directly linked to kidney disease.

In both examples (polypharmacy and comorbid conditions), the number and severity of dysfunctions is increasing which speeds up kidney disease progression.

We can't prove our theory of eliminating or reducing dysfunctions as the proper way to manage kidney disease to a clinical standard yet. We need more data, but I believe we will prove this to be true in the not too distant future. However, we can easily document that allowing the severity and number of dysfunctions to increase speeds up kidney disease progression and leads to worse outcomes for us.

Common sense would tell us reducing the number and severity of dysfunctions should benefit our overall health.

This is further evidence we need to address every aspect of our health and solve every dysfunction no matter how big or small. It doesn't matter if the condition is linked to kidney disease. We have to get 100% of the patient healthy, not just one part.

More pills and more diagnoses are the opposite of solving dysfunction at the root causes and lead to accelerated kidney disease and worse outcomes for us.

No matter how you look at this subject, dysfunctions, root causes, polypharmacy or comorbid conditions, we get the same evidence that reducing the number of dysfunctions (as we call them) is directly tied to your future health, quality of life, and rates of kidney and heart disease progression.

Chapter 11

Replacing Random Combinations With a Down-To-The-Milligram Approach to Dysfunctions

If we know our goal is to solve dysfunctions at the root cause while not creating any new dysfunctions, we have to come up with an approach that addresses all of the issues we face effectively and accurately. We have to manage all our problems simultaneously.

Some molecules build up in our system, others we excrete too much of, yet others we stop producing the right amount (hormones). We still need to get 100% of the recommended daily amounts (RDAs) for safe nutrition all while eliminating dysfunctions. Other issues like inflammation, oxidative stress, renal acid load, glycemic indexes, etc. also affect our future outcomes but are rarely measured—yet clearly matter.

How can we deliver the RDAs for safe and complete nutrition while trying to solve every possible dysfunction and bring everything back to normal? How can we lower nitrogen intake to get BUN levels back to normal or compensate accurately enough to improve GFRs? Protein restriction has been the primary tool in the past, but protein restriction is only one part of a much bigger dysfunctional picture.

The most overlooked problem of past kidney diets

When you start doing the nutritional math, trying to solve every dysfunction, follow current best practices and meet RDAs, a clear problem emerges in the first 60 seconds.

It's still mind-boggling to me that this problem has never been published or addressed before Kidneyhood.org started because it is so obvious when you start trying to solve real problems.

One incredibly overlooked aspect of kidney diets and related nutrition is that **everything was developed in isolation** from each other. In many cases, each component was developed in a different country, different decade and different manufacturer and never meant to be combined or used together.

Each part of the diet or dietary combination was developed in isolation and with no knowledge of the other's ingredients, content, goals, or even existence. None of the components—the diet plan, the keto acid analog or protein supplement, the vitamins, etc.—were clinically proven to be effective individually or in combination with each other.

It's no one's fault, everyone was working with what they had at the time, but the problem still stands. Random combinations are the exact opposite of accurate compensation for diseased kidneys or solving dysfunctions. It's likely impossible for random combinations to have a measurable effect on our health or kidney disease progression. We see this in study after study.

The outcome is that no kidney diets combination so far has demonstrated the ability to slow disease progression rates to lower-than-normal rates or return BUN levels back to the normal ranges.

If we are being critical, the use of random and unproven combinations of diets, medical foods, and or supplements does not pass even the slightest scrutiny when the argument is framed correctly or if we take the time to do the nutritional math to calculate nitrogen loads, check against best practices, or ensure RDAs are met.

Based on decades of data, we decided to take a different approach and do the opposite of previous approaches to kidney disease.

Doing the math leads to integration as the answer to randomness and solving real dysfunctions.

When we started the Kidneyhood.org project, we did the math and concluded it was 100% impossible to thread this very precise needle using random combinations. We also knew that the nitrogen content of keto acid analogs would have to be much lower than in past options to achieve normal BUN levels.

We also found it was 100% impossible to follow current best practices and achieve RDAs by combining random things. Every kidney diet has nutritional shortfalls and excesses, which have to be planned for and dealt with effectively. There is no way around this fact. Many diets contribute to as many dysfunctions as they solve, so we get nowhere in real life.

The only possible solution is integrating everything to accomplish our goals.

If we care about RDAs, solving dysfunctions at the root cause, best practices and so on, there is only one possible solution. Every aspect of the kidney diet must be integrated to meet our larger goals of solving as many dysfunctions as possible (and all at once) while ensuring safety and nutrition. We have to replace randomness with down-to-the-milligram exactness when our kidneys are not functioning properly and cross-check everything to ensure we are not contributing to new dysfunctions.

We have to control our intake accurately enough to return blood tests back to the normal ranges and reduce wastes to a level our current kidney function can handle. If we can compensate accurately enough, we should be able to bring our tests back to the normal ranges or close. The best part is that no guessing is required, our blood and urine tests are the gold standard of information.

A secondary issue also has to be addressed. Kidney disease management is often counterintuitive, causing even the most well-intentioned attempts to fail.

One of the most daunting facts related to kidney disease is that so many aspects of our disease are counterintuitive or part of a complex set of relationships. Many of these complexities are still poorly understood making things even harder. Before going into the results, I want to give you a few examples of why kidney disease diets should be followed to the letter or as a *prescribed diet* as we call it sometimes. By a *prescribed diet* we mean following a specific diet exactly to the letter without substituting or changing anything, just like a prescription medication. This means every patient must be on the same diet. Think of a drug trial, they don't give patients hundreds of variations of the drug, everyone gets the same drug and in similar amounts to arrive at a clinically significant outcome. The same guideline should apply to kidney diets. When kidney diets are customized or changed, so is the outcome. Customizing diets is the road to hell if we are trying to achieve clinically significant outcomes. In our survey, the bottom 10% of patients (in terms of outcomes) all made up their own diets. The patients had good intentions, but kidney disease is complex and counterintuitive as you will see.

Every dietary or nutritional choice has both intended and unintended consequences that may change how your kidney disease progresses. We are always much more worried about the unintended consequence, and you should be too.

Albumin as an example of counterintuitive issues

Albumin is the most common protein in your bloodstream. When albumin levels start falling, everyone says to eat more protein. Falling albumin levels is a genuine cause for concern (not panic) and is a sign of oxidative stress, high acid loads, and/or potential protein nutrition issues.

On the surface, eating more protein makes sense. If a protein on your blood test is going lower, then eat more protein. We see this recommendation almost daily despite all evidence to the contrary. Adequate protein intake is required, but that is only part of the picture.

First, albumin is made by the liver, so it's not a direct dietary intake issue. Eating more protein will only help if you are protein deficient in some way. Second, eating more protein increases blood urea nitrogen (BUN), which in turn increases oxidative stress and inflammation and, eventually, lowers albumin levels. Albumin is so linked to oxidative stress that albumin is considered a biomarker for, or measure of, oxidative stress.

Third, eating more dietary protein increases acid load on your kidneys. Every 25 mEq/day increase in acid load was associated with decreasing albumin levels, and kidney disease progressed faster.[93] Increasing protein intake increases acid load, but lowering protein intake reduces acid load.

Because we don't fully understand our dysfunctions and these complicated and often counterintuitive relationships, we scar more nephrons and accelerate kidney disease progression by eating more protein in an attempt to increase albumin levels.

The opposite of conventional wisdom is required to improve albumin in many cases, and even then, it's still very hard to improve, and it takes time. We need to dramatically lower dietary protein intake to reduce blood urea nitrogen back to the normal range while providing the RDAs for each of the 9 essential amino acids. We also need to reduce oxidative stress by increasing antioxidant intake from real foods (not supplements) and reduce acid loads by going to a more alkaline (plant-based low or very low protein) diet. We need to do *everything all at once* to improve albumin levels. Only when we address the multiple factors that are lowering albumin can albumin start to rise or even stabilize. This approach also lowers the amount of albumin (protein) in your urine, so you are keeping more albumin in your blood which also helps in increasing albumin levels.

Does meeting current guidance or best practices matter?

While counterintuitive issues have to be dealt with successfully, valid fears also exist with regards to malnutrition or, in our case, many times overnutrition (too much of a good thing) drives progression.

One question we asked is: What is the best nutrition for kidney patients? Do we even know? Has it ever been defined?

The 2020 KDOQI is the closest thing we have to a quality control reference or agreement of experts about what nutrition should be.[1] KDIGO does not cover individual vitamins and minerals.

However, again, when you do the nutritional math, you will find in 60 seconds that it has been 100% impossible for us to follow current guidance in the past. This translates to it being 100% impossible for us to get modern healthcare from a nutritional point of view.

The truth is no one really knows what the actual intake of essential amino acids, nitrogen, vitamins, and minerals is on different program combinations when everything is added together (dietary + supplement intake).

We can debate whether this is a limiting factor or not in slowing kidney disease, but most of us can agree that we should be getting adequate nutrition and following modern, up-to-date best practices. Malnutrition is a common dysfunction and fear among kidney patients, so this must also be addressed.

Could you actually follow or follow the most up-to-date nutritional guidance?

Putting both essential amino acid recommendations and KDOQI-listed vitamin and mineral recommendations together leads to at least 179 calculations per day, assuming 3 meals/day and 3 foods with each meal. If you add in snacks or drinks, the number of daily calculations is well over 200/day.

You would have to spend hours calculating everything and then try to compensate for shortfalls or excesses. If you tried to do this on your own, you would have 20+ supplement bottles stacked to the ceiling and be trying to cut each pill or capsule to the appropriate amount, if needed at all. Who does this? You guessed it: no one, but this is what would be required to actually follow current guidance.

The only possible way to even get close to the goal of following current guidance and ensuring all nutritional goals are met, but not greatly exceeded, is an integrated approach where everything is designed to work together and every milligram is accounted for. All the work is done for patients using this model. We want to achieve our goals of complete nutrition and best practice compliance while addressing as many dysfunctions as possible including malnutrition and or overnutrition.

A prescribed diet designed to solve as many dysfunctions as possible combined with a custom keto acid analog and a custom, low-dose or low-serving-size vitamin all have to be developed in unison to work together in order to achieve any measure of accurate compensation. This way everything can be controlled down to the milligram, and we can ensure best practices and dysfunctions are managed appropriately. This is the only chance we have of accurate compensation for diseased or damaged kidneys.

Making it easy on patients to improve success rates and comply with modern best practices

Using an integrated approach where everything has already been calculated makes it easier on the patient. The Kidneyhood.org diet is designed to provide everyone with complete nutrition as long as they stay within the prescribed diet. No numbers need to be calculated daily. The only exception is if we are troubleshooting some very specific issue that did not resolve in the first 90 days. Most patients (80%–85%) never need help troubleshooting when everything is done for them. Success rates appear to be much higher using this approach.

Putting it all together at home

When we take a down-to-the-milligram approach to dysfunctions and root causes, follow modern best practices, ensure RDAs are met, and provide an exact dietary approach in which everything is integrated to work together, then and only then can patients realistically expect to be successful at home (on their own). We replace random combinations with precision, accuracy and modern best practices.

Dramatic improvements can be achieved at home by patients with no knowledge or limited knowledge of kidney disease, best practices, RDAs, etc. when we do the work for them.

By following an integrated program consisting of a prescribed diet with custom-made keto acid analogs and a custom low-dose multivitamin, a patient at home can do the following:

- Follow applicable best practices from KDOQI
- Follow applicable best practice from KDIGO
- Achieve RDAs for every essential amino acid
- Achieve RDAs for vitamins and minerals
- Follow a clinically proven program to reduce the number of dysfunctions
- Objectively evaluate effectiveness in 90 days or less using blood/urine tests
- Correct or change diet over time in response recent test results

This is a huge step up from the random, unproven combinations of the past and the practice of patients constructing their own diets with no idea if they are being successful or not. In terms of healthcare quality, this approach is a giant leap forward.

Everyone wins with this approach; patients and clinicians alike know they are following best practices and meeting RDAs, and results can be objectively evaluated over short periods of time using blood and urine tests.

Chapter 12

Early Data From Taking a Dysfunction, Damage and Best Practices Approach to Kidney Disease Management

Stages of studies

One of our major goals is to improve the quality of healthcare for kidney patients, so we opted to follow the drug model as a guide or blueprint for providing clinical effectiveness. We copied much of the drug testing processes to ensure effectiveness and validate everything we do. Our work is in patient education, nutrition, diet, and lifestyle—not drugs, to be clear. The drug model gives us a framework for proving or disproving diets or dietary combinations.

We also understand we are carrying 50 years of questionable results from past kidney diets on our back whether we like it or not. We are going to have to do multiple studies and trials to prove effectiveness to a clinical standard. It's going to take a lot of proof and evidence before any dietary approach will be accepted as a viable alternative for managing kidney disease.

The drug model

New drugs usually go through many steps. First, research is done with molecules in test tubes, then new drugs go through safety studies. If the drugs are successful, they move on to clinical studies or trials. Clinical research normally has 4 phases.

1. Phase 0 involves very few patients with a small dose of the drug to be tested.

2. Phase I is when 10–100 volunteers try the drug; the researchers are testing safety and dosage.

3. Phase II gives the drug to a few hundred people with the disease to see if it is effective and what side effects may occur.

4. Phase III is when many people (up to 3,000) first try the drug. After that, the FDA decides if the drug is safe enough to go to market.[94,95]

In the Kidneyhood.org model, stage 0 is me. I test everything and act as the head guinea pig for everything we do. I am always testing some improvement or variation to the program. My wife worries I am going to take this too far someday. I have had kidney disease for 25+ years and am still going strong against all odds. Being a human guinea pig has been pretty good to me.

I can tell you that 99% of the things I have tried did not move my blood/urine tests by a measurable amount. I have tried many things over 25 years from around the world. One improvement has shown promise over the current program, and we are working on testing this in 2025. We hope this change will make the program more effective. Our work on proteinuria and improving albumin are also ongoing, but it is proving to be very tough to get consistent results for every patient. We are gaining on this every year, but they are tough issues.

Stage 1 used actual before-and-after blood tests to be objective. We did not use patient surveys or opinions as evidence, only actual blood and urine tests. This was our first-year attempt to validate effectiveness with a group of volunteers in our program. We wanted to make corrections at this stage if we found problems. All (100%) patients submitting blood and urine tests improved in stage 1.

Stage 2 has closed as we were able to prove clinical effectiveness with fewer participants than expected. Results are later in this chapter for complete transparency. The next study is on GFR trajectories or trends over 2–5 years while trying to document the number of dysfunctions before and after. We still need to determine if this is the real driver of improvements like we theorize.

Stage 3 is in the future, and we will need a large institution or organization to help us due to the size of these studies. We will be ready for stage 3 once improvements to the program are put into practice. If you are with one of these large institutions or organizations, please email or call us as we are ready, willing, and able to cooperate with any study or trials. Evidence to date is that we can prove clinical effectiveness with a very small study size.

Please reach out to us at support@kidneyhood.org.

Results from a damage and dysfunctions approach to kidney disease

Before going over the results, I think it's important to stress again that these are early results, and we need larger studies to confirm. Any results you get will depend on dietary compliance, stage of kidney disease, overall health, etc. The FDA has not evaluated any statements here. Anyone who has spoken with me knows I try to be honest and cautious as a fellow patient. I would call our studies *emerging evidence* at this stage.

I would view these results as a range of what's possible given a serious integrated approach to kidney disease management using the dysfunction, damages, and best practices theory. It's an approach that reflects a modern, integrated, down-to-the-milligram model for kidney disease management as opposed to past random combinations. We had a few big questions going in. If we replaced randomness with a precision, down-to-the-milligram approach, ensured RDAs were met, and followed modern best practices, would we get better results? Could we solve more dysfunctions at the root cause? We would need to get greatly improved outcomes to prove random combinations were a key part of past failures.

You can view full study data in the Kidneyhood.org Pilot Study on page 133.

The dietary combination used in Kidneyhood.org studies

This is important to discuss as even small changes can change outcomes. When you change a single component or alter any dietary approach, nutritional intake and, therefore, outcomes will change.

The studies were based on the following integrated combination. All 3 components are needed to ensure nutritional goals and RDAs are met without patient calculations or changes. If you change or alter any one component, the results may change.

1. The **Kidneyhood.org diet** published as the Stopping Kidney Disease Food Guide. This book contains instructions and recipes for what would be considered a very low protein diet averaging 0.4 g/kg/day of dietary protein. If the diet is followed as designed, then all nutritional goals will be met when combined with Albutrix and Microtrix. Sixteen different factors are considered with intake increased or decreased by the predicted effect on dysfunctions or the ability to normalize blood tests. This diet was also designed with diabetics in mind and is low to medium on the glycemic index.

2. **Albutrix S3, S4 and S5** are **low nitrogen keto acid analogs** that were custom formulated based on the amounts of each of the 9 essential amino acids found in the foods in the diet plan. When dietary intake and Albutrix intake are totaled, the intake of essential amino acids meets the RDAs for each essential amino acid with the lowest possible nitrogen loads. The nitrogen content of the Albutrix series is just 190 mg—a 70% reduction in nitrogen intake compared to past keto acid analogs. Albutrix is also optimized for each stage of kidney disease. Daily intake of Albutrix is calculated to be 0.4 g/kg of body weight. (When added to protein intake from food, this meets the RDA for protein of 0.8 g/kg.) A secondary goal was increasing intake of potential protective keto acid analogs which has also the desired side effect of lowering nitrogen intake.

3. **Microtrix low serving multivitamin** is formulated specifically to supplement the prescribed diet. If intake from food is adequate, then the nutrient is not supplemented. For example, if we estimate that 70% of the RDA for Vitamin E comes from foods in the Kidneyhood.org diet, then only 30% of the RDA should be supplemented with Microtrix. It should be noted that no reputable kidney-related organization recommends high doses or servings of vitamins for patients not on dialysis, so a low-serving or low-dose multivitamin is needed.

All 3 integrated components (diet plan, keto acid analog, and multivitamin) are needed to make up any complete diet or nutritional strategy. The fourth component is a strong patient education program to ensure patients can be successful at home with little to no supervision. All patients in the study used all 3 components and had access to free coaching and troubleshooting for dietary issues.

If you change the diet, Albutrix, or Microtrix you have the potential for malnutrition and or the potential to change the outcomes.

For more information on this approach; Albutrix S3, S4, or S5; or Microtrix, please visit www.kidneyhood.org.

Our equivalent of Stage 1 data from patient volunteers

In our first year, we asked patients to submit results of before and after blood tests to determine if we were on the right track or not.

Seventeen patients responded with before and after blood test results. (Thank you to those early volunteers.)

Results were as follows:

+27% average increase in GFR/eGFR

-42% reduction in BUN levels with 80% of patients achieving normal BUN levels.

-25% reduction in creatinine levels.

Early results were already beating any published kidney diet data. Results were good enough to move on to our equivalent of a stage 2 study.

Stage 2: A formal study with 30 patients

This study was written to institutional review board (IRB) standards, but it has the weaknesses of not having a control group and small size. Despite the small size, we still met the drug standard for clinical effectiveness (*p*-values explained later) which is very exciting. To be clear, our program is not a drug or related to drugs, but we modeled our investigations after the drug standards because they offer a proven path to evaluate clinical effectiveness. For comparison, we can use other kidney diet study results instead of a control group. I am listing individual results for this study as I think it's more educational, and you can find someone with a similar GFR or BUN level to see what is possible. Thank you Dr. Alyssa Middleton for her help as clinical coordinator.

eGFR/GFR

How much can eGFR/GFR be improved with a dysfunctions, damage and best practices integrated approach over the short term?

Short term GFR improvements first

The first set of numbers only includes the baseline test and the next blood test that took place 2–6 months after the baseline test. This is the toughest criteria as we are looking for a statistically significant and measurable improvement in a very short period of time.

Baseline GFR	Next texts (2-6 months)	% increase/decrease
33.00	44.00	33.33%
20.00	19.00	-5.00%
20.51	25.57	24.67%
33.00	33.00	0.00%
10.00	11.00	10.00%
16.00	26.00	62.50%
26.00	40.00	53.85%
41.00	57.00	39.02%
35.00	41.00	17.14%
50.00	49.00	-2.00%
16.00	14.00	-12.50%
37.00	60.00	62.16%
16.00	35.00	118.75%
45.00	47.00	4.44%
35.51	47.20	32.92%
55.00	52.00	-5.45%
25.00	67.00	168.00%
51.00	47.00	-7.84%
32.00	44.00	37.50%

50.00	56.00	**12.00%**
38.00	40.00	**5.26%**
28.00	26.00	**-7.14%**
59.00	60.00	**1.69%**
27.00	28.00	**3.70%**
30.00	34.00	**13.33%**
22.00	25.00	**13.64%**
55.00	53.00	**-3.64%**
15.00	15.00	**0.00%**
12.00	14.00	**16.67%**
58.00	65.00	**12.07%**
38.00	42.00	**10.53%**
33.19	**39**	**Average +18.25%**

Based on a sample size of $n = 30$, GFR increased by an average of 18.25%. The increase in GFR was statistically significant (p <0.0001).

P-values (shown as $p < 0.0001$) are a calculation used to determine statistical significance or to ensure the results were not random or by chance. The lower the p-value, the more significant the finding or less likely that the outcome was random. P-values below 0.05 are considered clinically significant, and the same p-values standards are used for the drug approval process.

All measured aspects of our program (GFR, BUN, and creatinine) met the standard for being significant or *clinically proven*. This is the first time a published kidney diet has achieved this milestone to our knowledge.

Now, let's look at the highest GFR achieved over the next 6 months to 2 years. This gives us an idea of the maximum GFR gains over time.

Baseline GFR	Highest GFR over the next year	% increase/decrease
33.00	**55**	**66.67%**
20.00	**27**	**35.00%**
20.51	**33.41**	**62.90%**
33.00	**39**	**18.18%**

10.00	28	180.00%
16.00	30	87.50%
26.00	53	103.85%
41.00	57	39.02%
35.00	41	17.14%
50.00	63	26.00%
16.00	28	75.00%
37.00	60	62.16%
16.00	35	118.75%
45.00	60	33.33%
35.51	47.2	32.92%
55.00	60	9.09%
25.00	67	168.00%
51.00	53	3.92%
32.00	46	43.75%
50.00	64	28.00%
38.00	51	34.21%
28.00	34	21.43%
59.00	62	5.08%
27.00	28	3.70%
30.00	36.58	21.93%
22.00	25	13.64%
55.00	53	-3.64%
15.00	15	0.00%
12.00	20	66.67%
58.00	65	12.07%
38.00	55	44.74%
33.19	**44.87**	**Average 46.16%**

Based on a sample size of $n = 30$, GFR increased by an average of 46.16%. The increase in GFR was statistically significant ($p < 0.0001$).

Only 2 patients did not improve GFR over a longer time frame, but 1 did hold their GFR stable without dropping any GFR points. The group overall had a significant average improvement of over 40%. **We can document that the Kidneyhood.org program is very accurately compensating for our reduced kidney function.** We know that patients can improve for 12–24 months in a row. Big gains in the first 3 months and slow steady gains over the next months–years.

Varying levels of dietary compliance led to different results. We interviewed many of the patients, and even with less than perfect (50%–75%) self-rated dietary compliance, we found double-digit percentage improvements were still happening (9%–20% improvement in GFR). The most serious patients improved GFR by 50%+.

The most important question

GFR trajectory has improved dramatically and consistently for the first time. It's very clear now that combining random and unproven combinations was a driving factor in past failures to prove diet effectiveness. The reason is random combinations will never equal very accurate compensations for reduced kidney function or solve dysfunctions at the root cause. We have good data to show that we are solving dysfunctions at the root causes as most blood work returns to normal or continues to improve over time.

We are still trying to establish what is possible and best practices for the program as we go forward and collect more information. We are still learning and in the early stages. What we have established is that the GFR trajectory is improving dramatically within 90 days to 6 months on the Kidneyhood.org program, and these gains are being maintained with a flat-ish GFR slope anywhere from 2–5 years out.

GFR charts are a great educational tool.

Longer term data give us a window into what is happening over time with these patients. I wanted to include 3 charts, 1 extremely positive change, 1 more average outcome, and 1 outcome when changes were not as good. This will give us a more balanced view of what is possible and realistic.

Example 1: GFR going from 10–40 over 3 years

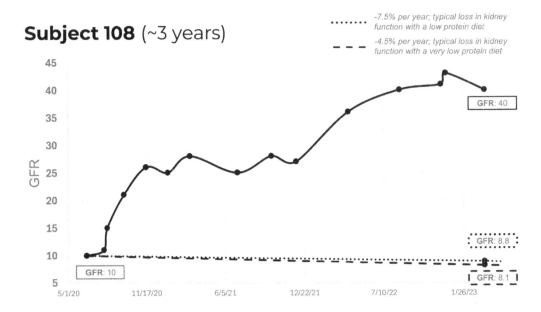

The patient in example 1 is an 84-year- old. The starting GFR was 10 mL/min/1.73 m² and the ending GFR was 40 mL/min/1.73 m² three years later. Starting blood urea nitrogen (BUN) level was 53 mg/dL, but BUN levels were reduced to the teens or well within the normal ranges (6–24 mg/dL). BUN levels dropped over 80%, but this was needed to achieve normal BUN levels.

Starting creatinine was 3.86 mg/dL and ending creatinine was 1.3 mg/dL or just at the top of the normal range. Normal creatinine range for this patient was 0.7–1.3 mg/dL. Again, we needed a very large drop in creatinine levels (70%+ reduction) to achieve normal creatinine levels.

This patient's blood work 3 years out looks like a normal healthy person for the most part despite being in their 80s with stage 5 kidney disease. He has gone from very sick needing imminent dialysis to looking much healthier from a blood test perspective.

Reducing BUN levels by 80%+ and improving creatinine levels by 70% doesn't happen by accident for someone with kidney disease.

We can easily document how accurately we have compensated for diseased kidneys. This patient is an extreme outlier, and these kinds of gains should not be expected, but these gains do illustrate what happens when we dramatically reduce the number and severity of dysfunctions at the root cause.

The patient changed diet and lifestyle and learned how to manage kidney disease and was rewarded with gains in health and GFR that are not supposed to be possible using past kidney disease management concepts.

Example 2: GFR rising from 20.51–29 over 4 years, 4 months

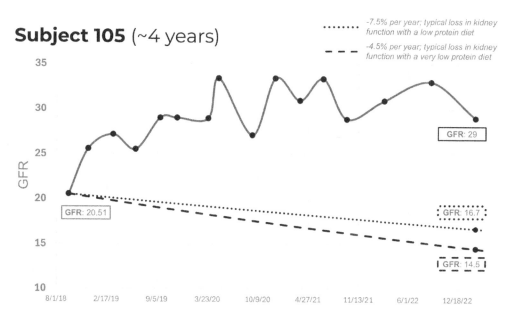

This patient was also in their 80s, but came into the program with less severe dysfunctions, so health gains are not as dramatic. The reason for less dramatic gains (we theorize) is that we did not reduce as many dysfunctions in both number and severity. Other reasons may exist, but this is where the data are pointing. This patient came into the program with BUN levels of 32 mg/dL that dropped to 23 mg/dL by the end of the period (normal range). Creatinine did not achieve normal ranges, but improved (2.3–1.74 mg/dL). From our viewpoint, the dysfunction of creatinine was not corrected, but was reduced in severity.

However, the patient's GFR is still 40% higher than the starting value after a little over 4 years with the program. Overall numbers are greatly improved, but not all tests made it back to the normal ranges.

Example 3: What it looks like when patients struggle with diet and lifestyle changes

This patient in the next example (and most of us) may struggle with dietary compliance or sticking with the prescribed diet (Kidneyhood.org program). I think it's a great example to give us a better understanding of how we improve or maybe don't improve. It also documents why we have to stick with these programs and not stop and start these diets. We need to make these changes semipermanent in most cases.

This patient started with a GFR of 16 mL/min/1.73 m^2 and had a GFR of 17 mL/min/1.73 m^2 18 months later. When troubleshooting dietary compliance, BUN levels are the first thing we look at. In this case, BUN levels started at 32 mg/dL and ended at 31 mg/dL, so very little changed. This tells us that protein intake was largely unchanged or slightly increased during the study period, despite the patient reporting dietary compliance with a very low protein diet. Creatinine also rose slightly from 2.95–3.00 mg/dL during the 3-year period. This patient's outcome was not that different from normal disease progression. We can also see that when blood tests come back worse, most patients will become more compliant with the diet in the short term. When the patient's GFR dropped to 14 mL/min/1.73 m^2, they became more compliant with diet for some time. GFR improved to 17–19 mL/min/1.73 m^2; a 25%–30% increase in GFR during this time. However, GFR gains fade over time when dietary compliance fades as well.

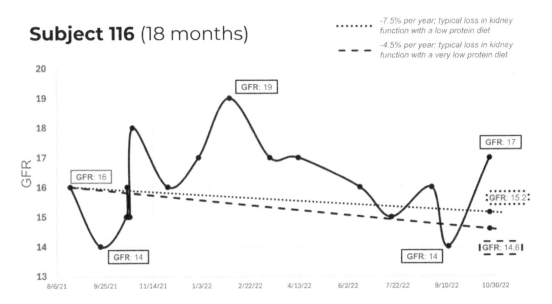

When we look at the blood tests, we can see that no dysfunctions were really solved or reduced dramatically. Based on the dysfunctions model, we would not expect much improvement and that is exactly what happened. If we don't solve any dysfunctions or improve our overall health, then we can't expect to have potentially life-changing outcomes.

Blood urea nitrogen

Now, let's look at blood urea nitrogen levels (BUN) for improvements across all people in the study. The normal range for BUN is 7–24 mg/dL in the US. Our goal was to achieve BUN levels in the normal ranges to short-circuit all of the dysfunctions related to high BUN levels.

BUN Baseline	After Kidneyhood.org program	Reduction in BUN levels
33.00	23.00	-30.30%
42.00	30.00	-28.57%
32.00	24.00	-25.00%
35.00	15.00	-57.14%
53.00	24.00	-54.72%
44.00	13.00	-70.45%
28.00	12.00	-57.14%
20.00	8.00	-60.00%
28.00	13.00	-53.57%
18.00	6.00	-66.67%
32.00	41.00	-28.13%
36.00	9.00	-75.00%
80.00	9.00	-88.75%
23.00	7.00	-69.57%
81.00	11.00	-86.42%
9.00	16.00	77.78%
27.00	16.00	-40.74%
24.00	13.00	-45.83%
28.00	27.00	-3.57%
11.00	9.00	-18.18%
25.00	19.00	-24.00%
23.00	9.00	-60.87%
27.00	28.00	3.70%
28.00	16.00	-42.86%
89.00	54.00	-39.33%
25.00	10.00	-60.00%
34.65	17.77	Average -51.28%

Based on a sample size of n = 26, BUN decreased by an average of 16.8 points or over 50% reduction in BUN levels. The decrease in BUN was statistically significant ($p <$ 0.0001).

For the first time in any published study, the average patient achieved normal BUN levels despite starting BUN levels being well outside the normal ranges. We have 2 sets of data now with BUN levels dropping from -42% to -51.28% and the vast majority of patients achieving normal BUN levels.

Achieving normal BUN levels is a huge success and gives us a precise guide to the exact right combination of dietary protein intake and keto acid analog nitrogen content. We know exactly what works to bring BUN levels back to the normal ranges now. With most patients achieving normal BUN levels, the current approach is about right in terms of dietary protein intake at 0.4 g of protein per kg of body weight per day. This is a 25%–33% increase in protein intake compared to the 0.3 g/kg used in traditional very low protein diets (VLPD+KA). Results were much better due to integration of diet and Albutrix. Again, getting rid of the random combinations that have so many unknowns and excesses was clearly part of the solution. The dramatically lower nitrogen content of Albutrix compared to most keto acid analogs allowed patients to have increased dietary protein intake and still achieved much higher reductions in BUN levels. A win-win for patients. We can expect approximately 80% of patients to achieve normal BUN levels based on past results. In medicine any treatment program with an 80% success rate would be considered very successful.

Patients achieving normal BUN levels would be expected to have a much better future outcome than those patients whose BUN levels are outside the normal range. We have moved a known driver of kidney and heart disease progression back to the normal range by going after the root cause of high BUN levels. **BUN levels as high as 80 mg/dL can be brought back to the normal ranges which has never been achieved prior to the Kidneyhood.org study.**

Creatinine

We have not talked much about creatinine in this book so far, but out-of-range creatinine levels are a common problem for patients. Creatinine is not as strong a predictor of future outcomes as GFR and BUN. Rising average creatinine levels happened on all diets (LPD, VLPD+KA, LPD+KA and plant-based diets) in most studies.

Creatinine levels are the hardest to improve because they are based mostly on muscle breakdown, which happens daily regardless of dietary intake. Diet-related issues do affect creatinine levels,but by a smaller amount.

Normal serum creatinine numbers are 0.7–1.3 mg/dL (61.9–114.9 μmol/L) for men and 0.6–1.1 mg/dL (53–97.2 μmol/L) for women.

I am showing the first and last creatinine test results in the chart below. The time difference from the first and the last creatinine test varied from 90 days to over two years depending on how much the patient submitted. I am listing all results for transparency and education on what is possible in terms of creatinine reductions. .

Creatinine Baseline	After Kidneyhood.org program	Creatinine reduction %
1.96	1.35	-31.12%
2.22	2.13	-4.05%
2.30	1.74	-24.35%
2.20	2.1	-4.55%
3.86	1.28	-66.84%
3.35	1.94	-42.09%
2.13	1.35	-36.62%
1.30	1.21	-6.92%
1.50	1.44	-4.00%
2.95	3	1.69%
1.75	1.24	-29.14%
3.57	2.28	-36.13%
1.53	1.17	-23.53%
1.40	1.3	-7.14%
1.45	1.35	-6.90%
2.92	1.28	-56.16%
1.41	1.61	14.18%
2.00	1.47	-26.50%
1.80	1.4	-22.22%
2.71	2.27	-16.24%
1.02	1.02	0.00%
2.09	2.43	16.27%
2.20	1.7	-22.73%
2.20	2.2	0%
1.26	1.32	4.76%

3.54	**3.39**	**-4.24%**
4.74	**3.12**	**-34.18%**
1.13	**1.02**	**-9.73%**
2.01	**1.5**	**-25.37%**
2.22	**1.75**	**Average -21.53%**

Creatinine levels dropped an average of -11% on the first blood tests and averaged a -23.7% reduction over longer terms. This is very similar to our stage 1 study with a -29% reduction in creatinine levels.

Again, lowering creatinine tells us we are solving real problems and more effectively compensating for our diseased kidneys. It is thought that the higher the creatinine, the lower the odds of success on kidney diets. This may or not be true for our program; we can't say for sure yet. However, even patients with creatinine levels above 5 mg/dL were able to improve.

Overall health versus just restricting protein

What we can see is that patients are very accurately and effectively compensating for damaged kidneys based on all 3 traditional measures of kidney function: GFR, BUN, and creatinine. We also see that other blood tests are improving at the same time. Issues like albumin and blood sugars are also stable on the integrated program.

We are using a modern disease prevention model (like heart disease diets) to try to solve the maximum number of dysfunctions at the root cause while doing as much of the work as possible for patients. It takes a very specialized, targeted and integrated approach to offset all the dietary and nutritional issues we experience as kidney patients. We still have a long way to go, but we are on the right track based on early testing and patient results.

Chapter 13

Understanding the Potential Benefits and Limits of Kidney Diets

A chapter is needed to clarify a few issues after reporting study data. It's important to your education that you understand how the gains were achieved and what the limits of kidney diets are. I also want to answer some common questions about the Kidneyhood.org study in this chapter and discuss how the results might apply in certain situations.

Gains

Improvements in GFR, creatinine and BUN happened because we lowered the waste workload to a level our kidneys can better handle or process. As an example, if we reduce the waste workload on our kidneys by 50%–70%, we are going to get a big improvement in blood tests. If we reduce the workload by 5%, then no improvements will show on our blood tests. We saw this with results from diets in Part 2; no meaningful change occurred in any tests as waste workloads did not change, despite a perception that diet was changed.

Many patients feel kidney disease has been cured or definitively treated because of improvements. Sadly, this is not the case. Your actual kidney function is exactly the same as before. Nothing has been healed or cured. Dialysis offers a good comparison. Dialysis does not attempt to cure kidney disease in any way. Dialysis is a treatment to remove or normalize excesses in our bloodstream. If these excesses are allowed to accumulate, we will die in a few weeks. Dialysis allows us to live for years with minimal kidney function by successfully managing excesses.

Dialysis is a form of kidney disease management, not a kidney disease cure.

Successful diets are methods of managing kidney disease, not curing the disease.

GFR, both unreliable and extremely accurate

Let's assume your diet is constant each year, then any changes in GFR would be an accurate indicator of your current kidney function. However, when we dramatically reduce the workload on your kidneys, GFR increases. If we can change GFR by changing dietary intake, then GFR is not an accurate indicator of our current kidney function or disease progression. If we go back to old dietary habits, then test results go right back to baseline. If we stop compensating for reduced kidney function, we lose the benefits. Dialysis has the same effect of improving GFR by reducing the amount of waste products in our bloodstream.

However, GFR or changes in GFR are a very accurate indicator of the waste workload or changes in waste workloads relative to your current kidney function. For this reason, long term dietary intake can be managed very accurately and effectively. If your GFR is not improving on your new diet, then you know you have not reduced the waste workloads enough to change your future outcome.

If your new improved GFR after dietary changes is holding steady, four to five years later we can assume your kidney function is holding steady as well. You are losing fewer nephrons in this example. Stable kidney function for years to come is our goal.

The very meaningful goal of normal

Our goal is *normal* blood tests, blood pressure, body weight, etc. Normal is where disease progression should be the slowest as there should be the fewest number of dysfunctions driving disease progression.

Successful kidney diets are methods to manage the excesses and shortfalls associated with reduced kidney function. We are managing these issues by reducing or increasing intake to reach normal ranges in our blood despite reduced kidney function. The same is true of nutrition. We need to eliminate or reduce risks of malnutrition by managing intake.

This quote from a study on 1,486 patients noted the following:[96]

"Analysis revealed that estimated glomerular filtration rate did not decline in patients who had a good achievement rate [met goals like normal blood tests, healthy weight, etc.], but decreased significantly in patients with a poor achievement rate [didn't meet the same health goals]."

Basically, those patients who were able to improve aspects of their blood tests did not show a decline in kidney function, but those who did not improve these issues lost GFR at a much faster rate. This is a very important fact. Different studies in this book have documented no meaningful progression of kidney disease over one year when everything is done right. We still don't understand everything , but multiple studies suggest that very slow or almost no measurable progression may be possible if we address enough dysfunctions at the root cause.

Limitations

Dialysis and kidney diets have similar limitations. They are not cures, and hormone and enzyme production is normally not affected by dialysis or kidney diets. Vitamin D, blood cell production hormone (erythropoietin), and blood pressure regulation enzyme (renin) levels are not improved by much. Our kidneys are still damaged and producing less of these hormones or enzymes. Neither approach can correct every issue associated with kidney disease.

How long can improvements last?

We don't know at this point. Our data extends to 5 years, so we only know it's at least 5 years. A few very early adopters are still going strong and very close to the 6-year mark.

How low can GFR be when starting to manage kidney disease with diet?

This will depend greatly on the dietary approach used. The record-holder here started with a GFR of 6 and delayed dialysis by 3 years before needing it after a major surgery. What we see in real life is that patients who start the program with a GFR around 10 or below eventually go on dialysis at some point. The reason for dialysis has normally been a major surgery or illness combined with already very low kidney function. These patients have been sick for a long time and have normally accumulated several comorbid or other health issues.

We normally recommend a GFR of 12 as the absolute minimum for starting a kidney diet to have a realistic chance of improvements or delaying dialysis. We would normally add about 25% to your GFR as an estimate of potential gains. If you start when your GFR is 10 and get a 25% gain, you are still in dialysis territory with a GFR of 12.5. Starting with a GFR of 12 only gets us to a GFR of 15, but that is starting to get out of dialysis territory.

I also want to make clear these diets are harder with lower GFRs. Dietary restrictions are harder when we have less kidney function to work with. More restrictions and more tweaking of diet is needed when GFRs are this low. The earlier you start, the easier it will be as you will have more kidney function to work with. *Don't wait* is my message here as you want to preserve as much kidney function as you can.

Do kidney diets work for every form of kidney disease?

We don't know. The majority of patients (75%+) never have a biopsy, so we never know what type of kidney disease we are fighting.

People with genetic diseases like polycystic kidney disease (PKD) appear to respond just like every other patient with improved numbers, but we don't know how these diets affect cyst growth. Is cyst growth the same, slower, or faster? No one knows the answer at this time, based on our review of current studies.

Autoimmune forms of kidney disease are also a mixed bag. Some patients reported extremely positive results, and others much more muted improvements. We don't have enough data to give an accurate opinion yet. These patients respond like everyone else, but we do not know how these improvements may affect the underlying autoimmune disease.

We will talk about how to deal successfully with so many variables on an individual level in the conclusion.

Chapter 14

What About Supplements?

I wanted to add this chapter before closing this book. Questions on supplements are second only to questions on vegan, vegetarian, or plant-based diets. Supplements pose a lot of problems for us as patients with limited kidney function. I just had a call with a gentleman taking 27 supplements, so this is a common issue we see.

No standards for effectiveness

The first hurdle we have is that as a group, supplements, foods, or even medical foods are not required to provide proof of effectiveness and many cannot be measured with a blood test. We have all seen how good these companies are getting at marketing, and marketing claims blur the lines so much that everything looks wonderful.

Just like diets, dietary advice, and diet books, supplements have no mandate or requirement to prove or disclose effectiveness, outcomes, risks, etc. Dietary advice is the least regulated part of the diet world, but supplements are a close second.

This matters because what we are finding is that even the most benign supplements may change our outcomes. Remember the probiotics example from the chapter on root causes. Cancer patients had worse outcomes taking probiotics compared to high-fiber diets.[78]

Excesses are part of the problem.

Excess intake leads to excess wastes or excess byproducts that our kidneys cannot eliminate fast enough. These excesses may build up in our body causing problems for us. Most, if not all, supplements are higher servings or doses when compared to the RDA, or in many cases, no RDA exists at all. In these cases, we don't know what is considered excess intake as no standard exists. We also don't know if excess intake contributes to excesses that can harm us.

You should strongly consider limiting any and all dietary supplements if you are a kidney patient unless prescribed by your doctor.

Some examples of excesses

High-dose or large serving niacin (vitamin B3) was used to lower cholesterol for some time, but then it was determined that niacin did not lower the risk of heart attack or stroke.[97] Now, byproducts of excess niacin breakdown called 2PY and 4PY are known causes of cardiovascular problems. People with 2PY or 4PY levels in the top 25% had 1.6–2 times the risk of major cardiac events over the next 3 years as those with levels in the bottom 25%, even after controlling for other cardiovascular risk factors.[98]

In general, high dose or serving B vitamins may lead to increased rates of kidney disease progression or increased rates of heart disease.[99]

Supplemental calcium may increase the risks of heart disease,[100] but dietary calcium is beneficial.

Excess vitamin D intake can cause kidney damage.

Excess iron intake can also cause kidney damage.

Fat soluble vitamins are more likely to build up in our system (Vitamin A, D, E and K).

High vitamin C intake can increase the risks of oxalates.

And many more.

We see the example again and again. The waste byproducts of excess intake are what seems to increase our risks, but normal dietary intake from real food does not. We need adequate intake to meet the RDAs, but not excess intake.

Less is more for kidney patients

We know excesses are not handled well by diseased kidneys, so why are we taking more than the RDAs or adequate intake? If we know excess intake is a problem, and the supplement is not clinically proven to improve our outcomes or recommended by your doctor, why are we taking unknown risks?

While patients may assume supplements are effective, physicians may assume every supplement is a scam because they are not clinically proven to be effective or change outcomes. Opposite opinions for identical products or supplements should raise another red flag for us.

From our early data, it appears patients who take the most supplements have the most variable or least predictable outcomes. Patients taking the fewest or no supplements appear to have much more predictable outcomes. The assumption is that some supplements or combinations of supplements are affecting outcomes in ways we don't yet understand. When outcomes don't match expectations, supplement review is part of the troubleshooting process due to the number of excesses and extremes created from supplement intake (normally very high servings or doses). When we eliminate or greatly reduce the number of supplements, results normally improve and become more consistent. We are trying to compile more data on this issue to better advise patients in the future even though this might be an impossible task due to the sheer number of supplements.

When patients are taking multiple supplements, the odds of excess intake go through the roof.

My message here is be conservative. Supplemental intake cannot be assumed to be benign or harmless.

Label research illustrates the problem we face

To drive this point home even further, the Clean Label Project, (an independent nonprofit organization that examines labeling safety issues) found that virtually all of the 134 products they tested contained detectable levels of at least one heavy metal, and 55% tested positive for Bisphenol A (BPA). BPA is a substance used in plastics manufacturing and is considered harmful.[101]

A 2010 Consumereports.org study similarly detected arsenic, cadmium, lead, and/or mercury in samples of all the 15 protein powders tested.[102]

Yet, another study found around 40% of the 57 supplements bought online did not contain a detectable amount of the ingredient listed. Half displayed the wrong amount, and 12% were found to contain illegal additives. Only 11% of products were accurately labeled according to this study.[103]

I do not want to imply that 100% of supplements are bad or harmful without exception. My point here is diets and dietary supplements represent the least regulated area and have so many unknown issues combined with normally excess intake. Be careful, deliberate and conservative with supplemental intake. You have to be your own guardrail and quality control. Excess intake is almost guaranteed with supplemental intake. Be careful out there and think of terms *only if* to reduce risks and unknowns.

Using the *only if* rule to limit or eliminate supplemental intake

The list of supplements or medical foods that can be considered recommended or proven for kidney diets is very short. What is important from a patient education standpoint is that each supplement or medical food is recommended _only if_ a certain condition is met.

No kidney- or health-related organization in history has ever recommended taking random amounts of anything or large serving sizes far in excess of the RDA.

Remember, we want to live in a world of modern science where safety and effectiveness are common.

In the 2020 KDOQI,[1] the following are recommended, and the advice is always conditional:

1. **Sodium bicarbonate** <u>only if</u> acidosis is an issue and not controlled by a low-acid or alkaline diet.

2. **Authentic or real keto acid analogs** <u>only if</u> on a very low protein diet or not meeting RDAs for protein/essential amino acids from dietary intake.

3. **Vitamin D** supplements <u>only if</u> vitamin D levels are below normal range.

4. **Long-chain Omega-3 polyunsaturated fatty acids** <u>only if</u> triglycerides are high.

5. **Supplementation of any vitamin/mineral**[5] <u>only if</u> blood tests show you are below the normal range or a known deficiency exists. The goal is to get you back into the normal range of everything. You must always know what dietary intake is or have blood tests to determine if supplementation is needed.

We could also add CoQ10 to the list as most patients are on statins, and CoQ10 was proven effective in other studies, but it was not covered in the 2020 KDOQI.[1,104] CoQ10 could be recommended *only if* you are taking a statin or cholesterol-lowering drug.

Start thinking in terms of *only if*.

We should copy the KDOQI recommendations and think in terms of *only if*. If we are not solving known problems or dysfunctions effectively, then there is no reason to take most supplements, vitamins, medical foods and so on. We could easily be creating more dysfunctions than we are solving or reducing the effectiveness of some other aspect of a dietary program.

What you don't see on the recommended list

What you don't see on this list of recommended supplements is just as important. You don't see herbal remedies, traditional supplements, high-dose vitamins, teas, ancient secrets, homeopathic cures, or any number of wild internet claims that get forwarded to us.

Your odds are always best with clinically proven treatments and/or options recommended by reputable organizations like the National Kidney Foundation (NKF), the

---

5   I am summarizing much of the KDOQI individual recommendations here.[1]

KDOQI, your physician, or diets and dietary combinations that have proof of clinical effectiveness and or adequate nutrition.

My message here is to be conservative in your approach to kidney disease and be very careful not to add to excesses and unknowns. Less is more with reduced kidney function.

Conclusion

Clinically Significant and Life-Changing Outcomes as Our Real Goal

In the introduction, I mentioned the mass confusion related to kidney diets. Patients and clinicians are unsure what works and what doesn't. We see evidence of confusion everywhere we look.

While kidney disease is systemic, complicated, counterintuitive and currently incurable in most cases, we can still answer many questions with the available data. We can greatly reduce the amount of confusion related to kidney diets by applying some objective standards that reflect our goals as patients.

We only need to guess if we are unwilling to look at the published evidence or if we don't know how to measure or evaluate these diets or dietary combinations.

Years of our lives are not small matters (at least to us)

The assumption in this book is that you want to change your future with kidney disease by a measurable amount. We patients are after life-changing outcomes compared to the normal progression rates of kidney disease. We don't want to improve a little; we want to improve dramatically. Slowing kidney disease progression even a little is beneficial, but not what we are really after as patients. We are after long, healthy, high-quality lives just like everyone else. Kidney disease management is already a difficult fight and made much harder than it has to be when so much confusion is allowed to exist.

We can eliminate over 99% of any confusion regarding kidney diet effectiveness by applying simple, but objective standards. We need *drug-like* objective standards to make a hard fight much easier and less confusing for us all.

The minimum standard for kidney/renal diets should be:

1. **GFR loss of less than -3% per year**

2. **The ability to return BUN levels to normal ranges.**

These two predictive measures represent the <u>bare minimum</u> needed to improve our future outcome with kidney disease compared to normal disease progression rates. Minimum standards give us easy and objective methods to reduce confusion that every patient and clinician has access to. Every dietary approach to kidney disease can be objectively evaluated in minutes using minimum standards. If you will apply these basic standards, you will eliminate 99% of the confusion related to kidney diets.

It's also important to understand no single diet or product proved effective on its own when the standard is slowing progression to rates slower than normal kidney disease progression. Diet alone won't work (no matter what the diet is) and keto acid analogs alone won't work either(no matter what keto acid analog is used) and supplements also have no record of achieving our goals. Only an integrated approach trying to eliminate as many dysfunctions as possible has the potential to achieve our goals in 2025.

Another way to look at what is most recommended is to consider what dietary approaches have demonstrated at least some potential to achieve our goals.

It's clear in 2025, VLPD+KA has the most potential. However, different variations will produce different outcomes, but some form of VLPD+KA is clearly where we must start. The available evidence also points to mostly plant based VLPD+KA.

We are not the only ones coming to this conclusion. The only dietary combination that both the KDIGO and the KDOQI agree on is very low low protein diets supplemented with keto acid analogs(VLPD+KA).

A reminder of how many people are behind these recommendations may help:

KDOQI- is a joint publication of the National Kidney Foundation and the American Academy of Nutrition and Dietetics . These recommendations were reviewed and contributed by over 40 researchers, dietitians, nutritionists and physicians.

KDIGO-The International Society of Nephrology publishes the KDIGO. The recommendations in the KDIGO were reviewed or contributed to by over 30 researchers, dietitians, nutritionists and physicians.

Over 70 researchers and physicians in the USA and EU came to the similar conclusions as this book. This is a very important fact from a quality control perspective.

In 2025, any approach to kidney disease must solve more problems than created and solve these problems decisively enough to meet the highest standards(like drugs). As patients, when we waste time on conflicting data or pursue approaches that have never been proven to work, we are wasting kidney function, time, energy, emotions and money.

It does take time and effort on our part, but I promise the benefits are worth the effort.

While there are no guarantees in our outcome and any changes or variations in dietary approach will change outcomes, we still have to determine what is best for us.

Rapid validation by being a guinea pig

Everyone's situation and health issues are a little different, and most patients don't even know what type of kidney disease they have (no biopsy). Some patients are willing to follow more strict diets to slow kidney disease progression and others are not. This makes it difficult, if not impossible, to determine what is best for each patient on an individual basis due to the thousands of potential combinations of stage of disease, type of disease, dietary compliance, comorbid conditions and so on.

Once we lose kidney function, we lose it forever. Therefore our goal is rapid validation or rapid invalidation to any approach to kidney disease management. Rapid validation of any dietary approach or dietary combination can be done despite so many unknowns and variables.

You can rapidly and objectively evaluate any dietary approach or combination by following the recommendations or diets faithfully without changes or substitutions in as little as 30 days. 30 days is a very short period of time, but you should be able to see small, but measurable improvements . 90 days is a better gauge or measure, but if you wanted to rapidly validate something, it could be done in 30 days.

If you try any dietary approach or dietary combination faithfully and follow the instructions or guidance without changing or substituting, after 30–90 days you will get an objective answer from your blood/urine tests; you won't have to guess about effectiveness. Your blood tests are the gold standard for information. **Our goal as patients is very rapid and objective evaluation despite so many variables.**

If you alter, substitute, change, or stray from the instructions or guidance and get less than stellar results, you won't know what caused the problems or poor outcomes. Garbage in, garbage out.

One issue you have seen repeatedly in this book is that small changes in dietary or supplemental intake also can change outcomes.

When I made the most progress, it was when I framed what I was doing as an objective experiment. I followed the plan to the letter to make my results objective instead of subjective. Clearly, I am a slow learner as it took me years of failure to start becoming more objective in my approach. I hope you can learn from my years of mistakes.

It should be possible now for most patients to achieve positive trajectories in GFR, reduce BUN levels back to the normal ranges and improve creatinine levels in a very short amount of time (30–90 days). This is very important because following the *guinea pig process is the* only way to objectively validate or invalidate any dietary program or approach. Rapid and objective evaluations give us tools to keep improving or changing until we get to something that does work for our situation. Rapid and objective evaluations also give us the tools to evaluate marketing claims compared to actual results.

We can't say for sure yet what is possible with the Kidneyhood.org program as we need a larger study to confirm, but if you approach any diets or dietary approach as a guinea pig for 30–90 days at time, you can determine exactly what works best for your current health and form of kidney disease.

If you are not achieving these meaningful health goals and normal ranges, it's time to rethink things or try a different approach. The early and emerging evidence from our program is very promising, but you still need to be an objective guinea pig to find out what works for you.

Being the most help a kidney patient has ever received.

This is the goal of Kidneyhood.org. We know how difficult it can be to live with kidney disease. Being confused, unsure and anxious is a daily thing for us especially after diagnosis of *incurable diseases*. My hope is this book will give you the data, education and evidence you need to dramatically change your future outcome with kidney disease like hundreds of other patients have.

Let factual, up-to-date, verifiable evidence replace internet garbage, scams, guessing, ignorance and a tremendous amount of old and outdated information.

Dietary management combined with drugs are the only logical approach at this time

I sincerely believe we are on the verge of dramatic improvements in both dietary and prescription drug options to slow and successfully manage kidney disease over decades. The reason for my optimism is so many aspects of kidney disease can only be managed through dietary intake and we are progressing rapidly in this area. Drugs cannot manage or eliminate many of the dysfunctions we normally experience as kidney patients. This means the combination of a dietary approach and drugs represents the only real route to dramatic and hopefully life changing outcomes. Kidney diets are incomplete without drugs like blood pressure medications and drugs are incomplete because they do not lower or control dietary intake. Our opinion is any serious approach to kidney disease management must use a combination of drugs and diets to solve the most dysfunctions possible. Any single approach will always be less effective.

Please take your health today and your future health seriously and take whatever steps are needed to ensure you're around for the next big breakthrough and for your family. You can live a high quality, active and pretty normal life despite having kidney disease.

Your education on kidney disease will be the biggest factor in your future outcome. I hope this book will dramatically reduce the amount of confusion regarding kidney diets and also expose you to new, emerging evidence that may be the biggest improvement in dietary kidney disease management in decades. Stay tuned.

Go guinea pigs!

Please reach out to us at www.kidneyhood.org or support@kidneyhood.org if we can help in any way.

References

1. Ikizler TA, Burrowes JD, Byham-Gray LD, et al. KDOQI clinical practice guideline for nutrition in CKD: 2020 update. *Am J Kidney Dis.* 2020;76(3 Suppl 1):S1-S107. doi:10.1053/j.ajkd.2020.05.006

2. Stevens PE, Ahmed SB, Carrero JJ, et al. KDIGO 2024 clinical practice guideline for the evaluation and management of chronic kidney disease. *Kidney Int.* 2024;105(4):S117-S314. doi:10.1016/j.kint.2023.10.018

3. Hilliard S, Tortelote G, Liu H, Chen CH, El-Dahr SS. Single-cell chromatin and gene-regulatory dynamics of mouse nephron progenitors. *J Am Soc Nephrol.* 2022;33(7):1308-1322. https://news.tulane.edu/pr/study-examines-why-kidneys-can't-regenerate-after-birth

4. Rai NK, Wang Z, Drawz PE, Connett J, Murphy DP. CKD progression risk and subsequent cause of death: A population-based cohort study. *Kidney Med.* 2023;5(4):100604. doi:10.1016/j.xkme.2023.100604

5. Kim JS, Hwang HS. Vascular calcification in chronic kidney disease: Distinct features of pathogenesis and clinical implication. *Korean Circ J.* 2021;51(12):961-982. doi:10.4070/kcj.2021.0995

6. Disthabanchong S. Vascular calcification in chronic kidney disease: Pathogenesis and clinical implication. *World J Nephrol.* 2012;1(2):43-53. doi:10.5527/wjn.v1.i2.43

7. Aoki J, Kaya C, Khalid O, et al. CKD progression prediction in a diverse US population: A machine-learning model. *Kidney Med.* 2023;5(9):100692. doi:10.1016/j.xkme.2023.100692

8. Writing Group for the CKD Prognosis Consortium, Grams ME, Coresh J, et al. Estimated glomerular filtration rate, albuminuria, and adverse outcomes: An individual-participant data meta-analysis. *JAMA.* 2023;330(13):1266-1277. doi:10.1001/jama.2023.17002

9. Grams ME, Sang Y, Ballew SH, et al. Evaluating glomerular filtration rate slope as a surrogate end point for ESKD in clinical trials: An individual participant meta-analysis of observational data. *J Am Soc Nephrol.* 2019;30(9):1746-1755. doi:10.1681/ASN.2019010008

10. Weng SC, Chen CM, Chen YC, Wu MJ, Tarng DC. Trajectory of estimated glomerular filtration rate and malnourishment predict mortality and kidney

failure in older adults with chronic kidney disease. *Front Med.* 2021;8:760391. doi:10.3389/fmed.2021.760391

11. Tsai CW, Ting IW, Yeh HC, Kuo CC. Longitudinal change in estimated GFR among CKD patients: A 10-year follow-up study of an integrated kidney disease care program in Taiwan. *PLOS ONE.* 2017;12(4):e0173843. doi:10.1371/journal.pone.0173843

12. Seki M, Nakayama M, Sakoh T, et al. Blood urea nitrogen is independently associated with renal outcomes in Japanese patients with stage 3-5 chronic kidney disease: A prospective observational study. *BMC Nephrol.* 2019;20(1):115. doi:10.1186/s12882-019-1306-1

13. Kim HJ, Kim TE, Han M, et al. Effects of blood urea nitrogen independent of the estimated glomerular filtration rate on the development of anemia in non-dialysis chronic kidney disease: The results of the KNOW-CKD study. *PloS One.* 2021;16(9):e0257305. doi:10.1371/journal.pone.0257305

14. Chen L, Chen L, Zheng H, Wu S, Wang S. The association of blood urea nitrogen levels upon emergency admission with mortality in acute exacerbation of chronic obstructive pulmonary disease. *Chron Respir Dis.* 2021;18:14799731211060051. doi:10.1177/14799731211060051

15. Duan S, Li Y, Yang P. Predictive value of blood urea nitrogen in heart failure: A systematic review and meta-analysis. *Front Cardiovasc Med.* 2023;10:1189884. doi:10.3389/fcvm.2023.1189884

16. Jiang S, Fang J, Li W. Protein restriction for diabetic kidney disease. *Cochrane Database Syst Rev.* 2023;1(1):CD014906. doi:10.1002/14651858.CD014906.pub2

17. Sohouli MH, Mirmiran P, Seraj SS, et al. Impact of low-protein diet on cardiovascular risk factors and kidney function in diabetic nephropathy: A systematic review and meta-analysis of randomized-controlled trials. *Diabetes Res Clin Pract.* 2022;191:110068. doi:10.1016/j.diabres.2022.110068

18. Chewcharat A, Takkavatakarn K, Wongrattanagorn S, et al. The effects of restricted protein diet supplemented with ketoanalogue on renal function, blood pressure, nutritional status, and chronic kidney disease-mineral and bone disorder in chronic kidney disease patients: A systematic review and meta-analysis. *J Ren Nutr.* 2020;30(3):189-199. doi:10.1053/j.jrn.2019.07.005

19. Li XF, Xu J, Liu LJ, et al. Efficacy of low-protein diet in diabetic nephropathy: A meta-analysis of randomized controlled trials. *Lipids Health Dis.* 2019;18(1):82. doi:10.1186/s12944-019-1007-6

20. Hahn D, Hodson EM, Fouque D. Low protein diets for non-diabetic adults with chronic kidney disease. *Cochrane Database Syst Rev.* 2020;10(10):CD001892. doi:10.1002/14651858.CD001892.pub5

21. Rhee CM, Ahmadi SF, Kovesdy CP, Kalantar-Zadeh K. Low-protein diet for conservative management of chronic kidney disease: A systematic review and meta-analysis of controlled trials. *J Cachexia Sarcopenia Muscle.* 2018;9(2):235-245. doi:10.1002/jcsm.12264

22. Patel J, Kalantar-Zadeh K, Joshi S. Low-protein diets and its synergistic role in the SGLT2 inhibitor era. *Adv Kidney Dis Health.* 2023;30(6):523-528. doi:10.1053/j.akdh.2023.12.005

23. Obeid W, Hiremath S, Topf JM. Protein restriction for CKD: Time to move on. *Kidney360.* 2022;3(9):1611. doi:10.34067/KID.0001002022

24. Jiang Z, Zhang X, Yang L, Li Z, Qin W. Effect of restricted protein diet supplemented with keto analogues in chronic kidney disease: A systematic review and meta-analysis. *Int Urol Nephrol.* 2016;48(3):409-418. doi:10.1007/s11255-015-1170-2

25. Yang W. The effect of the diet of nitrogen-free analogs of essential amino acids on chronic kidney disease deterioration: A meta-analysis. *Ther Apher Dial.* 2022;26(5):879-888. doi:10.1111/1744-9987.13795

26. Świątek Ł, Jeske J, Miedziaszczyk M, Idasiak-Piechocka I. The impact of a vegetarian diet on chronic kidney disease (CKD) progression - a systematic review. *BMC Nephrol.* 2023;24(1):168. doi:10.1186/s12882-023-03233-y

27. Dinu M, Colombini B, Pagliai G, et al. Effects of vegetarian versus Mediterranean diet on kidney function: Findings from the CARDIVEG study. *Eur J Clin Invest.* 2021;51(9):e13576. doi:10.1111/eci.13576

28. Garneata L, Stancu A, Dragomir D, Stefan G, Mircescu G. Ketoanalogue-supplemented vegetarian very low-protein diet and CKD progression. *J Am Soc Nephrol.* 2016;27(7):2164-2176. doi:10.1681/ASN.2015040369

29. de Mello VDF, Zelmanovitz T, Perassolo MS, Azevedo MJ, Gross JL. Withdrawal of red meat from the usual diet reduces albuminuria and improves serum fatty acid profile in Type 2 diabetes patients with macroalbuminuria. *Am J Clin Nutr.* 2006;83(5):1032-1038. doi:10.1093/ajcn/83.5.1032

30. Soroka N, Silverberg DS, Greemland M, et al. Comparison of a vegetable-based (soya) and an animal-based low-protein diet in predialysis chronic renal failure patients. *Nephron.* 1998;79(2):173-180. doi:10.1159/000045021

31. Burstad KM, Cladis DP, Wiese GN, Butler M, Hill Gallant KM. Effects of plant-based protein consumption on kidney function and mineral bone disorder outcomes in adults with Stage 3-5 chronic kidney disease: A systematic review. *J Ren Nutr.* 2023;33(6):717-730. doi:10.1053/j.jrn.2023.04.004

32. Valim A, Carpes LS, Nicoletto BB. Effect of vegetarian diets on renal function in patients with chronic kidney disease under non-dialysis treatment: A scoping review. *J Bras Nefrol.* 2022;44(3):395-402. doi:10.1590/2175-8239-JBN-2021-0126

33. Amir S, Kim H, Hu EA, et al. Adherence to plant-based diets and risk of CKD progression and all-cause mortality: Findings from the chronic renal insufficiency cohort (CRIC) study. *Am J Kidney Dis.* 2024;83(5):624-635. doi:10.1053/j.ajkd.2023.09.020

34. Piccoli GB, Capizzi I, Vigotti FN, et al. Low protein diets in patients with chronic kidney disease: A bridge between mainstream and complementary-alternative medicines? *BMC Nephrol.* 2016;17:76. doi:10.1186/s12882-016-0275-x

35. FoodData Central. Accessed August 11, 2024. https://fdc.nal.usda.gov/fdc-app.html#/food-details/172475/nutrients

36. Carrero JJ, González-Ortiz A, Avesani CM, et al. Plant-based diets to manage the risks and complications of chronic kidney disease. *Nat Rev Nephrol.* 2020;16(9):525-542. doi:10.1038/s41581-020-0297-2

37. Bellizzi V, Signoriello S, Minutolo R, et al. No additional benefit of prescribing a very low-protein diet in patients with advanced chronic kidney disease under regular nephrology care: A pragmatic, randomized, controlled trial. *Am J Clin Nutr.* 2022;115(5):1404-1417. doi:10.1093/ajcn/nqab417

38. Khor BH, Tallman DA, Karupaiah T, Khosla P, Chan M, Kopple JD. Nutritional adequacy of animal-based and plant-based Asian diets for chronic kidney disease patients: A modeling study. *Nutrients.* 2021;13(10):3341. doi:10.3390/nu13103341

39. Walser M, Hill SB, Ward L, Magder L. A crossover comparison of progression of chronic renal failure: Ketoacids versus amino acids. *Kidney Int.* 1993;43(4):933-939. doi:10.1038/ki.1993.131

40. Walser M, Hill S, Ward L. Progression of chronic renal failure on substituting a ketoacid supplement for an amino acid supplement. *J Am Soc Nephrol.* 1992;2(7):1178-1185. doi:10.1681/ASN.V271178

41. Masud T, Young VR, Chapman T, Maroni BJ. Adaptive responses to very low protein diets: The first comparison of ketoacids to essential amino acids. *Kidney Int.* 1994;45(4):1182-1192. doi:10.1038/ki.1994.157

42. Walser M, LaFrance ND, Ward L, VanDuyn MA. Progression of chronic renal failure in patients given ketoacids following amino acids. *Kidney Int.* 1987;32(1):123-128. doi:10.1038/ki.1987.181

43. Walser M, Thorpe B. *Coping with Kidney Disease: A 12-Step Treatment Program to Help You Avoid Dialysis.* 1st edition. Wiley; 2004.

44. Li A, Lee HY, Lin YC. The effect of ketoanalogues on chronic kidney disease deterioration: A meta-analysis. *Nutrients.* 2019;11(5):957. doi:10.3390/nu11050957

45. Ariyanopparut S, Metta K, Avihingsanon Y, Eiam-Ong S, Kittiskulnam P. The role of a low protein diet supplemented with ketoanalogues on kidney progression in pre-dialysis chronic kidney disease patients. *Sci Rep.* 2023;13(1):15459. doi:10.1038/s41598-023-42706-w

46. Milovanova L, Fomin V, Moiseev S, et al. Effect of essential amino acid ketoanalogues and protein restriction diet on morphogenetic proteins (FGF-23 and Klotho) in 3B-4 stages chronic kidney disease patients: A randomized pilot study. *Clin Exp Nephrol.* 2018;22(6):1351-1359. doi:10.1007/s10157-018-1591-1

47. Chang G, Shih HM, Pan CF, Wu CJ, Lin CJ. Effect of low protein diet supplemented with ketoanalogs on endothelial function and protein-bound uremic toxins in patients with chronic kidney disease. *Biomedicines.* 2023;11(5):1312. doi:10.3390/biomedicines11051312

48. Chang JH, Kim DK, Park JT, et al. Influence of ketoanalogs supplementation on the progression in chronic kidney disease patients who had training on low-protein diet. *Nephrology (Carlton).* 2009;14(8):750-757. doi:10.1111/j.1440-1797.2009.01115.x

49. Sánchez-Martínez C, Torres-González L, Alarcón-Galván G, et al. Anti-inflammatory and antioxidant activity of essential amino acid α-ketoacid analogues against renal ischemia-reperfusion damage in Wistar rats. *Biomédica.* 2020;40(2):336-348. doi:10.7705/biomedica.4875

50. Chen HY, Sun CY, Lee CC, et al. Ketoanalogue supplements reduce mortality in patients with pre-dialysis advanced diabetic kidney disease: A nationwide population-based study. *Clin Nutr Edinb Scotl.* 2021;40(6):4149-4160. doi:10.1016/j.clnu.2021.01.045

51. Lin YL, Hou JS, Wang CH, Su CY, Liou HH, Hsu BG. Effects of ketoanalogues on skeletal muscle mass in patients with advanced chronic kidney disease: Real-world evidence. *Int J Food Sci Nutr.* 2021;91-92:111384. doi:10.1016/j.nut.2021.111384

52. Klahr S, Levey AS, Beck GJ, et al. The effects of dietary protein restriction and blood-pressure control on the progression of chronic renal disease. *N Engl J Med.* 1994;330(13):877-884. doi:10.1056/NEJM199403313301301

53. KDIGO 2017 clinical practice guideline update for the diagnosis, evaluation, prevention, and treatment of chronic kidney disease–mineral and bone disorder (CKD-MBD). *Kidney Int Suppl.* 2017;7(1):1-59. doi:10.1016/j.kisu.2017.04.001

54. Yang C, Shi X, Xia H, et al. The evidence and controversy between dietary calcium intake and calcium supplementation and the risk of cardiovascular disease: A systematic review and meta-analysis of cohort studies and randomized controlled trials. *J Am Coll Nutr.* 2020;39(4):352-370. doi:10.1080/07315724.2019.1649219

55. Chang LL, Rhee CM, Kalantar-Zadeh K, Woodrow G. Dietary protein restriction in patients with chronic kidney disease. *N Engl J Med.* 2024;390(1):86-89. doi:10.1056/NEJMclde2304134

56. Vanholder R, Argilés A, Baurmeister U, et al. Uremic toxicity: Present state of the art. *Int J Artif Organs.* 2001;24(10):695-725.

57. Stenvinkel P, Alvestrand A. Inflammation in end-stage renal disease: Sources, consequences, and therapy. *Semin Dial.* 2002;15(5):329-337. doi:10.1046/j.1525-139x.2002.00083.x

58. Kaur G, Singh J, Kumar J. Vitamin D and cardiovascular disease in chronic kidney disease. *Pediatr Nephrol.* 2019;34(12):2509-2522. doi:10.1007/s00467-018-4088-y

59. Appel LJ, Brands MW, Daniels SR, et al. Dietary approaches to prevent and treat hypertension: A scientific statement from the American Heart Association. *Hypertension.* 2006;47(2):296-308. doi:10.1161/01.HYP.0000202568.01167.B6

60. Kraut JA, Madias NE. Metabolic acidosis of CKD: An update. *Am J Kidney Dis.* 2016;67(2):307-317. doi:10.1053/j.ajkd.2015.08.028

61. Block GA, Klassen PS, Lazarus JM, Ofsthun N, Lowrie EG, Chertow GM. Mineral metabolism, mortality, and morbidity in maintenance hemodialysis. *J Am Soc Nephrol.* 2004;15(8):2208. doi:10.1097/01.ASN.0000133041.27682.A2

62. Kittiskulnam P, Johansen KL. The obesity paradox: A further consideration in dialysis patients. *Semin Dial*. 2019;32(6):485-489. doi:10.1111/sdi.12834

63. Felsenfeld AJ, Levine BS, Rodriguez M. Pathophysiology of calcium, phosphorus, and magnesium dysregulation in chronic kidney disease. *Semin Dial*. 2015;28(6):564-577. doi:10.1111/sdi.12411

64. Maroz N, Simman R. Wound healing in patients with impaired kidney function. *J Am Coll Clin Wound Spec*. 2013;5(1):2-7. doi:10.1016/j.jccw.2014.05.002

65. Beier K, Eppanapally S, Bazick HS, et al. Elevation of blood urea nitrogen is predictive of long-term mortality in critically ill patients independent of "normal" creatinine. *Crit Care Med*. 2011;39(2):305. doi:10.1097/CCM.0b013e3181ffe22a

66. Tang Z, Yu S, Pan Y. The gut microbiome tango in the progression of chronic kidney disease and potential therapeutic strategies. *J Transl Med*. 2023;21(1):689. doi:10.1186/s12967-023-04455-2

67. Zha Y, Qian Q. Protein nutrition and malnutrition in CKD and ESRD. *Nutrients*. 2017;9(3):208. doi:10.3390/nu9030208

68. Borrelli S, Provenzano M, Gagliardi I, et al. Sodium intake and chronic kidney disease. *Int J Mol Sci*. 2020;21(13):4744. doi:10.3390/ijms21134744

69. Afsar B, Kiremit MC, Sag AA, et al. The role of sodium intake in nephrolithiasis: epidemiology, pathogenesis, and future directions. *Eur J Intern Med*. 2016;35:16-19. doi:10.1016/j.ejim.2016.07.001

70. Teucher B, Dainty JR, Spinks CA, et al. Sodium and bone health: impact of moderately high and low salt intakes on calcium metabolism in postmenopausal women. *J Bone Miner Res*. 2008;23(9):1477-1485. doi:10.1359/jbmr.080408

71. D'Elia L, Galletti F, Strazzullo P. Dietary salt intake and risk of gastric cancer. In: Zappia V, Panico S, Russo GL, Budillon A, Della Ragione F, eds. *Advances in Nutrition and Cancer*. Springer; 2014:83-95. doi:10.1007/978-3-642-38007-5_6

72. Gupta DK, Lewis CE, Varady KA, et al. Effect of dietary sodium on blood pressure: A crossover trial. *JAMA*. 2023;330(23):2258-2266. doi:10.1001/jama.2023.23651

73. Chang AR, Anderson C. Dietary phosphorus intake and the kidney. *Annu Rev Nutr*. 2017;37:321-346. doi:10.1146/annurev-nutr-071816-064607

74. Kato K, Nakashima A, Ohkido I, Kasai K, Yokoo T. Association between serum phosphate levels and anemia in non-dialysis patients with chronic kidney disease: A retrospective cross-sectional study from the Fuji City CKD Network. *BMC Nephrol*. 2023;24(1):244. doi:10.1186/s12882-023-03298-9

75. Asghar MS, Avinash F, Singh M, et al. Associated factors with uremic pruritus in chronic hemodialysis patients: A single-center observational study. *Cureus*. 13(8):e17559. doi:10.7759/cureus.17559

76. Seliger S, Waddy SP. Chapter 29 - Neurologic complications of chronic kidney disease. In: Kimmel PL, Rosenberg ME, eds. *Chronic Renal Disease (Second Edition)*. Academic Press; 2020:441-461. doi:10.1016/B978-0-12-815876-0.00029-2

77. Cao C, Zhu H, Yao Y, Zeng R. Gut dysbiosis and kidney diseases. *Front Med*. 2022;9:829349. doi:10.3389/fmed.2022.829349

78. Spencer CN, McQuade JL, Gopalakrishnan V, et al. Dietary fiber and probiotics influence the gut microbiome and melanoma immunotherapy response. *Science*. 2021;374(6575):1632-1640. doi:10.1126/science.aaz7015

79. Cheng F, Li Q, Wang J, Wang Z, Zeng F, Zhang Y. The effects of oral sodium bicarbonate on renal function and cardiovascular risk in patients with chronic kidney disease: A systematic review and meta-analysis. *Ther Clin Risk Manag*. 2021;17:1321-1331. doi:10.2147/TCRM.S344592

80. FoodData Central. Accessed August 11, 2024. https://fdc.nal.usda.gov/fdc-app.html#/food-details/175040/nutrients

81. Parohan M, Sadeghi A, Nasiri M, et al. Dietary acid load and risk of hypertension: A systematic review and dose-response meta-analysis of observational studies. *Nutr Metab Cardiovasc Dis*. 2019;29(7):665-675. doi:10.1016/j.numecd.2019.03.009

82. Sodium bicarbonate interactions. Drugs.com. Accessed August 13, 2024. https://www.drugs.com/drug-interactions/sodium-bicarbonate.html

83. van Oosten MJM, Logtenberg SJJ, Hemmelder MH, et al. Polypharmacy and medication use in patients with chronic kidney disease with and without kidney replacement therapy compared to matched controls. *Clin Kidney J*. 2021;14(12):2497-2523. doi:10.1093/ckj/sfab120

84. Oosting IJ, Colombijn JMT, Kaasenbrood L, et al. Polypharmacy in patients with chronic kidney disease. *Kidney360*. Published online April 25, 2024. doi:10.34067/KID.0000000000000447

85. Okpechi IG, Tinwala MM, Muneer S, et al. Prevalence of polypharmacy and associated adverse health outcomes in adult patients with chronic kidney disease: Protocol for a systematic review and meta-analysis. *Syst Rev.* 2021;10(1):198. doi:10.1186/s13643-021-01752-z

86. Laville SM, Metzger M, Stengel B, et al. Evaluation of the adequacy of drug prescriptions in patients with chronic kidney disease: Results from the CKD-REIN cohort. *Br J Clin Pharmacol.* 2018;84(12):2811-2823. doi:10.1111/bcp.13738

87. Wang X, Yang C, Jiang J, Hu Y, Hao Y, Dong JY. Polypharmacy, chronic kidney disease, and mortality among older adults: A prospective study of national health and nutrition examination survey, 1999-2018. *Front Public Health.* 2023;11:1116583. doi:10.3389/fpubh.2023.1116583

88. Shouqair TM, Rabbani SA, Sridhar SB, Kurian MT. Evaluation of drug-related problems in chronic kidney disease patients. *Cureus.* 2022;14(4):e24019. doi:10.7759/cureus.24019

89. Kimura H, Tanaka K, Saito H, et al. Association of polypharmacy with kidney disease progression in adults with CKD. *Clin J Am Soc Nephrol.* 2021;16(12):1797-1804. doi:10.2215/CJN.03940321

90. Tonelli M, Wiebe N, Guthrie B, et al. Comorbidity as a driver of adverse outcomes in people with chronic kidney disease. *Kidney Int.* 2015;88(4):859-866. doi:10.1038/ki.2015.228

91. Lee WC, Lee YT, Li LC, et al. The number of comorbidities predicts renal outcomes in patients with Stage 3–5 chronic kidney disease. *J Clin Med.* 2018;7(12):493. doi:10.3390/jcm7120493

92. MacRae C, Mercer SW, Guthrie B, Henderson D. Comorbidity in chronic kidney disease: A large cross-sectional study of prevalence in Scottish primary care. *Br J Gen Pract.* 2021;71(704):e243-e249. doi:10.3399/bjgp20X714125

93. Banerjee T, Sebastian A, Frassetto L. Association of diet-dependent systemic acid load, renal function, and serum albumin concentration. *J Ren Nutr.* 2023;33(3):428-434. doi:10.1053/j.jrn.2023.01.007

94. Office of the Commissioner. The Drug Development Process. FDA. February 20, 2020. Accessed March 24, 2024. https://www.fda.gov/patients/learn-about-drug-and-device-approvals/drug-development-process

95. Office of the Commissioner. Step 3: Clinical Research. FDA. April 18, 2019. Accessed March 24, 2024. https://www.fda.gov/patients/drug-development-process/step-3-clinical-research

96. Wang Y, Lee YT, Lee WC, Ng HY, Wu CH, Lee CT. Goal attainment and renal outcomes in patients enrolled in the chronic kidney disease care program in Taiwan: A 3-year observational study. *Int J Qual Health Care*. 2019;31(4):252-260. doi:10.1093/intqhc/mzy161.

97. Schandelmaier S, Briel M, Saccilotto R, et al. Niacin for primary and secondary prevention of cardiovascular events. *Cochrane Database Syst Rev*. 2017;6(6). doi:10.1002/14651858.CD009744.pub2

98. Ferrell M, Wang Z, Anderson JT, et al. A terminal metabolite of niacin promotes vascular inflammation and contributes to cardiovascular disease risk. *Nat Med*. 2024;30(2):424-434. doi:10.1038/s41591-023-02793-8

99. Wang AYM, Afsar RE, Sussman-Dabach EJ, White JA, MacLaughlin H, Ikizler TA. Vitamin supplement use in patients with CKD: Worth the pill burden? *Am J Kidney Dis*. 2024;83(3):370-385. doi:10.1053/j.ajkd.2023.09.005

100. Myung SK, Kim HB, Lee YJ, Choi YJ, Oh SW. Calcium supplements and risk of cardiovascular disease: A meta-analysis of clinical trials. *Nutrients*. 2021;13(2):368. doi:10.3390/nu13020368

101. Clean Label Project. *Protein Powder White Paper*. Accessed August 17, 2024. https://cleanlabelproject.org/protein-powder-white-paper/

102. Health risks of protein drinks. Consumer Reports. July 2010. Accessed August 17, 2024. https://www.consumerreports.org/cro/2012/04/protein-drinks/index.htm

103. Cohen PA, Avula B, Katragunta K, Travis JC, Khan I. Presence and quantity of botanical ingredients with purported performance-enhancing properties in sports supplements. *JAMA Netw Open*. 2023;6(7):e2323879. doi:10.1001/jamanetworkopen.2023.23879

104. Raizner AE, Quiñones MA. Coenzyme Q10 for patients with cardiovascular disease. *J Am Coll Cardiol*. 2021;77(5):609-619. doi:10.1016/j.jacc.2020.12.009

Kidneyhood.org Pilot Study

Easy-to-read study summary for patients

An Integrated Dietary Approach to Kidney Disease Management Shows Promising Results in Pilot Study

Baran Erdik, MD, MHPA
Sanjaya Chauhan, PharmD, MS
Alyssa Middleton, PHD

INTRODUCTION:

The Kidneyhood.org pilot study was designed to collect information about how people's health changes when using the Kidneyhood.org program (the SKD diet, Albutrix, and Microtrix). Our primary goal at this stage is to rapidly improve the program. The fastest and lowest cost way for us to gather data is from patients already on the program. A second pilot study is already underway to implement lessons from this study.

Past approaches to kidney/renal diets used combinations of unrelated diets and products with little-to-no documented success in slowing kidney disease progression. It is very unlikely that random combinations of unproven diets, medical foods, or supplements could have a meaningful effect on an incurable disease. The Kidneyhood.org study is one comparison between using non-integrated diets and products compared with a fully integrated approach to kidney disease management.

The Kidneyhood.org program integrates every aspect of dietary intake down to the milligram when possible. Every part of the program is designed to work together with another aspect of the program. The goal is to lower waste workloads on our already damaged kidneys as much as possible while achieving good nutrition. Good nutrition means meeting the RDAs set by diet experts for vitamins, minerals and supplying enough calories or energy in food.

Adequate compensation for diseased or damaged kidneys can be objectively evaluated using standard blood/urine tests.

METHODS:

Email invitations to participate in this study were sent to patients who had a minimum of a 6-month consistent history of ordering Albutrix and Microtrix. Over 25 volunteers were disqualified from the study due to improper use of the program or not following instructions for Albutrix S3, S4 and S5 use. This highlighted the importance of better and more detailed education as part of an improved version of the program.

The 31 volunteers who qualified for the study gave researchers a copy of their lab results from the time they first bought Albutrix, their lab results 6 months later, and their lab results 1 year later. They also answered questions about their height, weight, race, age, etc and essay-type questions about any health changes since starting the program, things they liked, and so on.

Statistical tests were used to compare any changes in the volunteers' labs at 6 months and 1 year to lab numbers at the beginning.

RESULTS:

This is the first dietary approach to document a measurable improvement in glomerular filtration rate (GFR).

Eighty percent of participants improved eGFR at both 6 months and 1 year.

Starting or baseline eGFR averaged 33.19.

The average GFR increase was 9.9 points or a 25%+ improvement in eGFR.

This is the first study to show normal blood urea nitrogen levels at the end of the study for most participants. This was true even when starting blood urea nitrogen levels were greater than 80 mg/dl.

Ninety-two percent of participants had reduced blood urea nitrogen levels with an average reduction of over 50%.

Over 80% participants achieved normal BUN levels.

Blood sugar (glucose) levels remained stable throughout the study. This was needed to confirm that the dietary approach, Albutrix and Microtrix, were safe and appropriate for diabetics and pre diabetics despite being lower in protein than most diabetic diets.

Creatinine was lowered in over 80% of patients at both 6 months and 1 year.

Albumin levels rose slightly during the Kidneyhood.org program. Stable and rising albumin levels are desirable. Albumin can be affected by many things, so this gives us a broader measure of oxidative stress, acidosis, adequate protein nutrition and other factors that affect albumin levels together.

Other relevant data:

Patient compliance was very good for a dietary approach. Over 75% of patients were able to follow the program and be compliant. The Kidneyhood.org program does as much of the work as possible for the patients, so no daily calculations are needed in most cases.

Gains in GFR and reductions in blood urea nitrogen are being maintained for periods up to 5 years. Each year we are adding to this data.

CONCLUSIONS:

We think it should be possible now for the majority of patients to improve GFR and achieve normal blood urea nitrogen levels. **Patients can clearly learn to successfully manage kidney disease at home with the right tools and education**.

No study is perfect and this study was no exception. Study limitations were small size and lack of control group. (There weren't that many people in the study, and all of them were doing the Kidneyhood.org diet.) Larger studies are needed to validate the program and make sure it does what we think it does. (These may involve volunteers being randomly assigned to either the Kidneyhood.org program or another treatment – something this study did not do.) Based on the history of past renal/kidney diets, the bar will be very high for proving effectiveness, and multiple studies will be needed. This study should be considered emerging evidence.

A combined approach is needed(diets and drugs)

Any serious approach to kidney disease management combines drugs (like blood pressure medications), changes in diet, and lifestyle changes. Many issues that increase the speed of kidney disease can only be changed by diet, not by drug therapies. For this reason, we believe any serious approach to kidney disease will be a "drugs and diets" approach. Leaving any health condition, out-of-range blood test, or comorbid condition untreated or unmanaged will normally make kidney disease get worse faster.

Please see **"The Evidence Based Guide to Kidney/Renal Diets"** for more information. Full study is attached.

Any questions or comments can be sent to support@kidneyhood.org.

Lee Hull

An integrated dietary approach to kidney disease management shows promising results in pilot study

Baran Erdik, MD, MHPA

Sanjaya Chauhan, PharmD, MS

Alyssa Middleton, PHD

INTRODUCTION

Chronic kidney disease (CKD), hallmarked by a glomerular filtration rate (GFR) of less than 60 mL/min/1.73 m² or other indicators of kidney damage, has a high global burden with incidence reported as up to 15% of the global population and is often unrecognized until advanced stages.[1] Globally, incidence has been rising, possibly attributable to increases in diseases that are the main causes of CKD in the developed world such as type 2 diabetes or hypertension. CKD is considered chronic, and all etiologies of CKD are considered progressive. Thus, the main goal of treatment is typically to slow the progressive loss of kidney function as well as delay the time until renal replacement therapy is started. Beyond the typical therapy with angiotensin-converting enzyme inhibitors as well as therapy aimed at the etiology, dietary factors within the context of CKD have been at the forefront of research, as the kidneys regulate numerous end products of dietary intake along with vitamins and minerals. Although the beneficial effects of dietary interventions, namely low-protein diets (LPDs), have been shown in the literature, the optimal approach is unknown, and some studies have demonstrated conflicting results leading to a lack of general recommendations to date sometimes owing to a lack of adherence. We have examined the effects of a standardized very low-protein diet supplemented with keto acid analogues as well as appropriate vitamin intake to match recommended dietary allowances (RDAs) in patients with CKD.

Kidneyhood.org diet (KD) is a "turn-key" LPD that includes keto acid analog low-nitrogen protein food Albutrix S3, S4, or S5 and Microtrix low-serving multivitamin. The KD is compliant with relevant 2020 KDOQI and 2024 KDIGO guidelines; both recommend very low-protein diets combined with keto acid analogs. Previous studies that have included keto acid analogs have typically used Ketosteril. However, Ketosteril contains 864 mg of nitrogen per daily dose compared with Albutrix with < 200 mg of nitrogen, enabling the patients to consume 5–8 g more of dietary protein for a total of 0.4 g of dietary protein per kg of body weight per day. This means, as an example, that an 80 kg adult can consume 32 g of protein per day compared with 24 g if on a LPD supplemented with Ketosteril. Another advantage of increase in allowance of daily protein owing to lowered nitrogen load from keto acid analog supplementation is the possibility of using whole foods, not just specialty low-protein foods typically made from starch, increasing patient satisfaction and compliance. Finally, the KD includes educational material and instructions for patients in the form of a book titled "Stopping Kidney Disease Basics," and the patients are able to contact the program for support via phone calls, emails, or similar methods 24/7. In general, most patients that finish the self-education aspects as well as consult with the program coordinators, spend a year or longer on the diet.

The pilot study had several objectives focused on efficacy and nutritional safety. The primary goal was to evaluate the impact of the KD intervention on GFR trajectories. A secondary aim was to determine the level of dietary protein or supplemental nitrogen restriction needed to normalize blood urea nitrogen (BUN) levels; a target not achievable through existing pharmacotherapy. Lastly, the study aimed to assess whether the integrated dietary approach met patients' nutritional needs. Ultimately, the KD intervention seeks to improve kidney function in CKD patients, a more ambitious goal than the traditional aim of merely improving some kidney related tests.

METHODS

The KD study was a retrospective, longitudinal analysis conducted among past KD participants. Email invitations were sent to individuals who had been using Albutrix and Microtrix for at least 6 months and had reordered these products at scheduled intervals, indicating regular use. The email invitation (Appendix A) invited participants to respond if they were interested in joining the study. Those who responded were assigned a study identification number and provided with instructions to access the HIPAA-compliant, secure webpage where the study questionnaire (Appendix C) was hosted.

The questionnaire collected demographic information and responses to open-ended questions about participants' experiences with the program and any health changes since starting the KD regimen. Participants were asked to collect all laboratory data from the time of their first purchase of Albutrix up to the present day, with the earliest lab results recorded as baseline data. Medical records could be uploaded to the secure platform or mailed to the study coordinator, who manually entered all data into a secure spreadsheet (Appendix D).

Thirty-one participants completed the questionnaire and submitted lab results for at least 1 baseline and 1 follow-up visit. As a token of appreciation, each participant received a $200 Visa gift card.

RESULTS

The analysis included a total of 31 participants at baseline. Thirty of these participants submitted records for at least 1 year. Demographics are presented in Table 1. Data was analyzed at both the 6-month and 1-year marks. The analysis focused on the areas that have the most effect on kidney function: serum albumin, estimated glomerular filtration rate (eGFR), serum creatinine, BUN, and blood glucose levels. Descriptive statistics for these parameters are summarized in Table 2.

Table 1. Demographics of the Participants at Baseline

Characteristic		All participants (n = 31)
Age, mean (SD), y		70.3 (12.5)
Sex	Male No. (%)	18 (58.1)
	Female No. (%)	13 (41.9)
BMI, mean (SD), kg/m^2		23.5 (3.1)
White race, No. (%)		27 (87.1)

Table 2. Descriptive Statistics of Kidney Function Lab Parameters

Parameters		No.	Mean (SD)	Range
Serum albumin, g/dL	Baseline	20	4.1 (0.6)	2.9–5
	6-Month	19	4.2 (0.6)	3.2–5
	1-Year	19	4.1 (0.5)	3.2–4.7
eGFR, mL/min/1.73 m^2	Baseline	31	33.2 (14.4)	10–59
	6-Month	30	41.5 (15.9)	15–67
	1-Year	30	43.1 (15.7)	16–67
Serum creatinine, mg/dL	Baseline	30	2.19 (0.91)	1.02–4.74
	6-Month	28	1.74 ±(0.63)	0.95–3.39
	1-Year	29	1.74 (0.63)	1.02–3.39
BUN, mg/dL	Baseline	28	33.9 (19.7)	9–89
	6-Month	25	18.1 (10.6)	7–52
	1-Year	26	19.7 (11.5)	7–52
Blood glucose, mg/dL	Baseline	30	93.9 (16.4)	61–135
	6-Month	29	95.3 (20.3)	71–169
	1-Year	28	94.2 (17.0)	76–143

Serum Albumin

Descriptive statistics for serum albumin showed a mean value of 4.1 g/dL at baseline, 4.2 g/dL at 6 months, and 4.1 g/dL at 1 year. Analysis of variance (ANOVA) results (Table 3) indicated no significant difference in serum albumin levels over time ($F = 0.062$, $p = .940$, $\eta^2 = 0.002$). Albumin levels were stable.

Table 3. ANOVA of Serum Albumin Values

Cases	Sum of squares[a]	Mean square	F test (df)	P value	η^2
Time	0.034	0.017	0.062 (2)	0.940	0.002
Residuals	15.215	0.277	(55)		
[a]Type III sum of squares.					

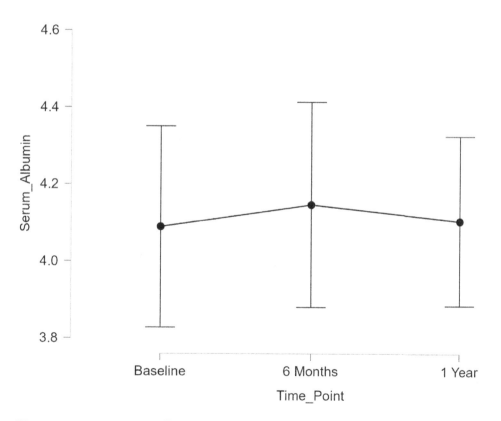

Figure 1. Mean serum albumin levels over time.

Estimated Glomerular Filtration Rate (eGFR)

The mean eGFR values were 33.2 mL/min/1.73 m^2 at baseline, 41.5 mL/min/1.73 m^2 at 6 months, and 43.1 mL/min/1.73 m^2 at 1 year. ANOVA (Table 4) revealed a significant difference over time ($F = 3.686$, $P = .029$, $\eta^2 = 0.077$). Post hoc analysis (Table 5) showed a significant increase in eGFR from baseline to 1 year (mean difference = 9.9, $P = .036$).

Table 4. ANOVA of eGFR Values

Cases	Sum of squares[a]	Mean square	F test (dF)	P value	η^2
Time	1741.781	870.891	3.686 (2)	.029	0.077
Residuals	20792.241	236.275	(88)		

[a]Type III sum of squares.

Table 5. Post Hoc Comparisons of eGFR Values by Time

		Mean difference	SE	t	P_{Tukey}[a]
Baseline	6 months	-8.3	3.9	-2.118	0.092
	1 year	-9.9	3.9	-2.521	0.036
6 months	1 year	-1.6	3.9	-0.400	0.916

[a]P value adjusted for comparing a family of 3.

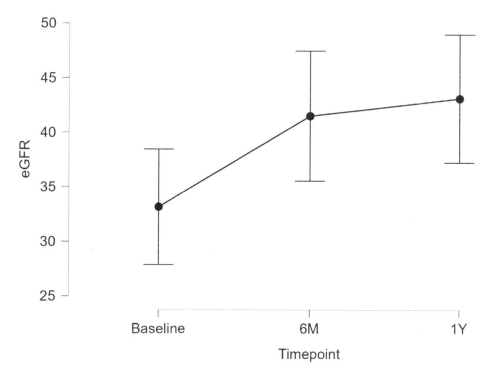

Figure 2. Mean eGFR levels over time.

Serum Creatinine

The mean serum creatinine levels were 2.19 mg/dL at baseline, 1.74 mg/dL at 6 months, and 1.74 mg/dL at 1 year. ANOVA (Table 6) indicated a significant reduction in serum creatinine levels over time ($F = 3.736$, $P = .028$, $\eta^2 = 0.080$). Post hoc comparisons (Table 7) showed a borderline decrease from baseline to 6 months (mean difference $= 0.45$, $P = .053$) and from baseline to 1 year (mean difference $= 0.45$, $P = .052$).

Table 6. ANOVA of Creatinine Values

Cases	Sum of squares[a]	Mean square	F test (dF)	P value	η^2
Time	4.058	2.029	3.736 (2)	.028	0.080
Residuals	46.705	0.543	(86)		
[a]Type III sum of squares					

Table 7. Post Hoc Comparisons of Creatinine Values by Time

		Mean difference	SE	t	P_{Tukey}[a]
Baseline	6 mo	0.45	0.19	2.359	0.053
	1 y	0.45	0.19	2.368	0.052
6M	1 y	-0.01	0.19	-0.011	1.000

[a]P-value adjusted for comparing a family of 3.

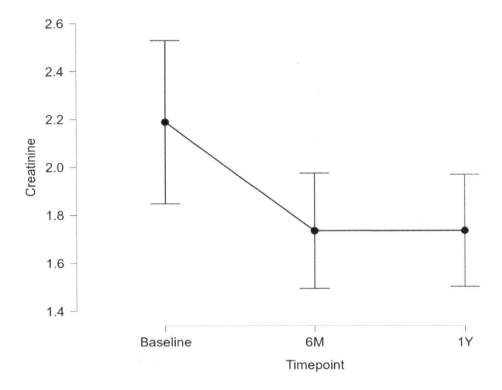

Figure 3. Mean serum creatinine levels over time.

Blood Urea Nitrogen (BUN)

The mean BUN levels were 33.9 mg/dL at baseline, 18.1 mg/dL at 6 months, and 19.7 mg/dL at 1 year. ANOVA showed a significant decrease in BUN levels over time ($F = 9.433$, $P < 0.001$, $\eta^2 = 0.199$). Post hoc tests (Table 9) revealed significant reductions from baseline to 6 months (mean difference = 15.8, $p = .001$, Cohens $d = 1.04$) and from baseline to 1 year (mean difference = 14.2, $P = .020$, Cohens $d = 0.89$).

Table 8. ANOVA of BUN Values

Cases	Sum of squares[a]	Mean square	F test (dF)	P value	η^{22}
Time	4083.042	2041.521	9.433 (2)	<.001	0.199
Residuals	16448.857	216.432	(76)		

[a]Type III sum of squares.

Table 9. Post Hoc Comparisons of BUN Results by Time

		Mean difference (95% CI)[a]	SE	t	P_{Tukey}
Baseline	6M[b]	15.8 (6.1-25.4)	4.048	3.896	<.001
	1Y	14.2 (4.6-23.8)	4.007	3.544	0.002
6M	1Y	-1.6 (-11.4 to 8.3)	4.121	-0.382	0.923

[a]P-value and confidence intervals adjusted for comparing a family of 3 estimates (confidence intervals corrected using the Tukey method).
[b]Abbreviations: 6M, 6 months; 1Y, 1 year.

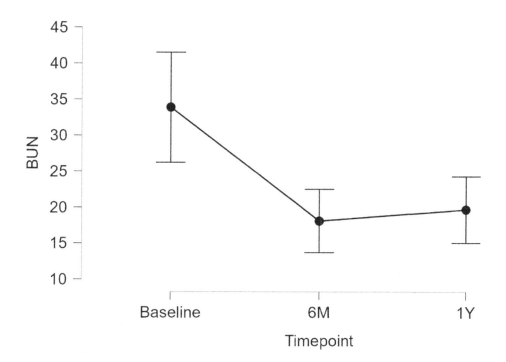

Figure 4. Mean BUN levels over time.

Blood Glucose

The mean blood glucose levels were 93.9 mg/dL at baseline, 95.3 mg/dL at 6 months, and 94.2 mg/dL at 1 year. ANOVA (Table 10) showed no significant change in blood glucose levels over time ($F=0.044$, $P=.957$, $\eta^2=0.001$).

Table 10. ANOVA of Blood Glucose Levels

Cases	Sum of squares[a]	Mean square	F test (dF)	P value	η^2
Visit	28.814	14.407	0.044 (2)	.957	0.001
Residuals	27198.910	323.797	(84)		
[a]Type III sum of squares.					

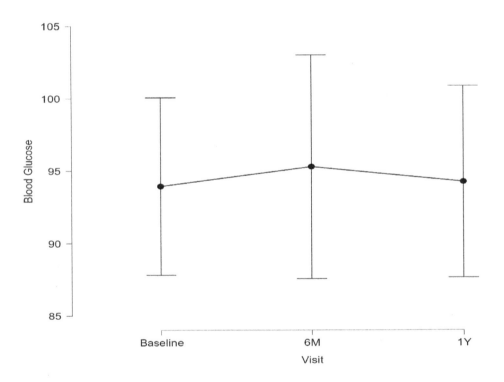

Figure 5. Mean blood glucose levels over time.

Change Summary Statistics

Eighty percent of participants had an improved eGFR at both 6 months and 1 year. Ninety-two percent had a decline in BUN at 6 months, and 84.6% still demonstrated this decline at 1 year. Serum creatinine decreased in 86.2% of participants at 6 months and in 83.3% of participants at 1 year.

The mean change in eGFR among participants in the Albutrix arm is 300% greater than the decline observed in historical data. Specifically, the mean change in eGFR in the Albutrix study was 9.9 mL/min/1.73 m^2, compared to a mean decline of about -5 mL/min/1.73 m^2 in the historical data.[2] This difference was statistically significant ($t = 6.951$, $df = 173$, $p < 0.001$), with a large effect size (Cohens $d \approx 0.93$), indicating that the Albutrix program led to a substantial clinical improvement in eGFR.

Qualitative Results

One open-ended question posed to participants was 'What Health-Related Changes Have You Noticed Since Starting the Stopping Kidney Disease Program?' Participants responded with a slew of positive health changes, which are summarized below along with some representative quotes.

- Significant improvement in GFR: "*...dialysis is not in my immediate future anymore*"

- Improved energy

- Improved digestive functions: "*no more heartburn*"

- Better workout stamina: "*not short of breath anymore*"

- Improved mental clarity

- More confidence

- Reduced the number of medications needed and/or medication dosage was reduced: "*Off all of my diabetes meds now*"

- Significant weight loss

- Improved mood (happier, more optimistic): "*I look and feel younger*"

- Less anxiety and stress "*not just about my disease being under control, but also about life in general*"

- Better cholesterol

- Increased libido

- Better sleep

- No more heart palpitations

Participants were effusive in their praise for the program. Some representative quotes include:

"The nephrologist is blown away! Initially he said the diet would not make a difference. Over the past three years her eGFR just steadily increased."

"It works! [Disease Management] requires a total commitment. No indication of nutritional issues on the food plan. Weight is holding for 1 year at 167, down from 212 before starting the program."

"With my current results, I am now very content and happy to stay with this program."

"Easy to follow."

DISCUSSION

LPDs have long been investigated in the management of CKD.[3] While early studies, particularly the landmark Modification of Diet in Renal Disease (MDRD) trial, failed to show definitive benefits, subsequent meta-analyses incorporating these data have consistently demonstrated the value of LPDs in slowing renal function decline and delaying dialysis initiation.[4,5] These findings align with physiological principles: reduced protein intake lowers urea production, diminishing the nitrogen load on kidneys. Urea, once considered inert, has now been implicated in insulin resistance, endothelial dysfunction, and atherogenesis, thus exacerbating CKD pathophysiology.[6,7]

Dietary protein induces hyperfiltration and glomerular damage, contributing to proteinuria, a marker and mediator of kidney injury. High-protein diets are linked to renal vasodilation, glomerular hypertension, and eventual glomerulosclerosis. In contrast, LPDs reduce hyperfiltration, particularly in diabetic nephropathy, by lowering proteinuria and mitigating glomerular damage. The additive benefit of LPDs complements the antiproteinuric effects of renin-angiotensin system inhibitors.[8-10]

Our study demonstrated significant improvements in key renal parameters. Estimated glomerular filtration rate increased by an average of 9.9 mL/min/1.73 m^2, while serum creatinine and BUN decreased significantly at both 6 months and 1 year when compared with historical data demonstrating a loss of 3.20 mL/min/1.73 m^2 for studies published after 2011, and when compared with 5.44 mL/min/1.73 m^2 for those published in the 1990s.[2] These changes are consistent with previous findings, highlighting the efficacy of standardized LPD interventions. In addition, plant-based diets, which have shown promise in CKD management, are believed to offer benefits through reductions in dietary phosphorus and acid load, as well as lower levels of indoxyl sulfate and other uremic toxins.[11] However, no single dietary approach including plant-based diets has been proven to improve eGFR or eGFR trajectories or achieve normal BUN levels.

One of the primary challenges to the success of LPDs has been adherence,[12] which can influence outcomes. Patient satisfaction was high with KD, with participants reporting improved health and a commitment to continuing the diet, despite initial skepticism from their nephrologists. In our study, the integrated support provided by Kidneyhood.org—offering continuous nutritional guidance and educational resources—resulted in a 75% adherence rate, a critical factor in the positive outcomes observed. The addition of keto acid analogs (KAs) further enhanced the benefits by reducing nitrogen load and preventing malnutrition, a common concern in LPD studies. KAs also demonstrated the ability to lower glomerular hyperfiltration and mitigate muscle catabolism, making them a valuable adjunct to LPDs.[13-15]

Conclusion

The primary objective of the KD was to reduce the nitrogen load on the kidneys through a standardized LPD while minimizing the risk of malnutrition. One of the most significant advantages of this approach is the demonstrated improvement in patient adherence, a critical factor that has compromised the outcomes of prior studies, including the MDRD trial. The KD program achieved high compliance rates by offering 24/7 support and standardized dietary guidelines, ensuring consistency in the approach. Our findings showed statistically significant reductions in creatinine and BUN, along with an increase in eGFR, aligning with numerous studies that affirm the benefits of LPD in CKD management.

A key difference between the KD program and previous studies lies in integration of all aspects of dietary intake. Most earlier studies were non-standardized, leading to inconsistent results due to variations in diet, KA supplementation, and patient adherence. The KD program's standardized approach mitigates these concerns, making it a scalable and easily reproducible solution that could significantly impact morbidity and mortality rates in CKD patients. From a public health perspective, slowing eGFR decline by even 1 mL/min/year could delay the need for dialysis, reducing both patient burden and healthcare costs. With a monthly cost of $200, the KD presents a cost-effective alternative to the expenses of dialysis.

Despite these promising outcomes, several limitations must be acknowledged. First, the patient cohort consisted solely of Stage 3 and 4 CKD patients who were not yet on dialysis, limiting the generalizability of the results to earlier stages of CKD.[16] While some studies suggest that earlier initiation of LPD may result in better long-term outcomes, this remains an area requiring further investigation.[17] Additionally, the KD program's success may be limited by the relatively small sample size and lack of randomization in our study. Although we demonstrated a statistically significant benefit, the underpowered nature of the study warrants cautious interpretation of the results. Future studies should aim for larger, more diverse populations with randomized, blinded designs to confirm the efficacy of LPDs in various CKD subtypes, especially in combination with KA supplementation.

Another consideration is the differential impact of LPDs on specific CKD etiologies. Diabetic nephropathy, for example, has shown the most benefit from protein restriction, whereas hypertensive CKD or polycystic kidney disease patients have demonstrated more modest results.[18] Thus, personalized dietary interventions may be necessary, further emphasizing the need for more detailed research. Finally, while our findings are encouraging, the retrospective nature of the study leaves room for potential confounders that may have influenced the observed improvements in renal function.

In conclusion, the KD program offers a standardized and scalable LPD with KA supplementation, which has demonstrated both safety and efficacy in reducing CKD progression. With further refinement and larger studies, the KD approach has the potential to become a key strategy in CKD management, addressing both clinical outcomes and public health challenges posed by the increasing global burden of CKD.

Appendix A

INITIAL EMAIL

Hello! Today I'm writing to invite you to participate in a current Kidneyhood.org study. We are looking to determine the results that customers have gotten after following the Stopping Kidney Disease diet and taking Albutrix / Microtrix, and asking for customer feedback on how we can improve.

Dr. Baran Erdik is our Principal Investigator, and he will oversee the study. We have a few others on our team as well, coordinating the day to day aspects of the study and analyzing the data. Rest assured that our team is experienced in conducting these types of studies and we have taken the necessary steps to ensure our study procedures and platform is HIPAA-compliant, meaning that your data is secure and everything will be kept confidential. Participants will be assigned an identification number. All results will be reported in aggregate, with no identifying information being shared.

It should take less than thirty (30) minutes to participate in this study. In exchange for your time completing the survey and submitting your lab reports, we will send a $200 Visa gift card to you.

If you're interested in being screened to see if you're eligible, or if you have any questions, please reply to this email or call Toni at (XXX) XXX-XXXX.

Thank you,

Lee Hull

P.S. If you don't want any more invitations to this research survey, click here.

Appendix B

EMAIL WITH PARTICIPATION INSTRUCTIONS

Dear (NAME),

Hello, thanks so much for your interest in participating in our study. This email provides information on how to access the survey and instructions. If at any time during the process you have questions, don't hesitate to call me at XXX-XXX-XXXX.

The link to access the study is: (LINK)

Your confidential study identification number is (ID#). You will need to enter your identification number on the first full page of the survey. .

Please read through the following instructions first, as you'll need to gather all of your information prior to accessing the survey.

Instructions to participate:

1. Gather bloodwork and urinalysis reports from the doctor's visit **closest to (DATE).** This will be considered your baseline visit. If you have a biopsy report, save that as well.

2. Then gather bloodwork and urinalysis reports from the rest of your doctor's visits from then until now. These will be approximately every 90 days or 3 months.

3. Scan and save these documents to your computer, ensuring the scans capture the date and all lab results on the image. It will be easiest for you if you save the documents as 'Baseline lab', 'Baseline urine', 'Visit 1 labs', etc so you can easily find them on your computer and ensure they are being uploaded correctly.

4. Go to the study website (LINK) and enter your subject identification number (ID#).

5. Complete the brief demographic questionnaire.

6. Click on 'Upload' next to Baseline labs. This will prompt your computer to search for the needed file. Select the correct document and hit 'Enter' on your keyboard. This will upload the document to the database.

7. Repeat these steps for all remaining documents to be uploaded.

8. Complete the final section of the questionnaire and provide feedback on the Stopping Kidney Disease diet and Albutrix.

9. When you are finished, click 'Submit'.

After we have confirmed all data has been uploaded, we will send you the $200 Visa gift card.

Should you prefer to mail your medical records to us so we can upload them for you, please mail them to:

There will be a checkbox in the survey for you to indicate that you have mailed the documents and will not be uploading them at that time.

If you have any questions, please reply to this email, or call me ,I'm happy to help you however I can.

Sincerely,

Dr. Alyssa Middleton

Kidneyhood.org

Appendix C

QUESTIONNAIRE

SECTION 1: DEMOGRAPHICS

1. Subject ID #
2. Date Started SKD Program
3. Age
4. Gender
5. Ethnicity/Race
6. List of medications and supplements (up to 10 spaces)
7. Diagnoses besides Chronic Kidney Disease (open text box)
8. Surgeries since starting the SKD program (open text box)
9. Weight prior to starting the Stop Kidney Disease diet
10. Current weight
11. Height
12. Most recent blood pressure reading
13. Have you had COVID-19 since starting the SKD program? (yes/no)

SECTION 2: UPLOADS

14. Biopsy report
15. Baseline blood work
16. Baseline urinalysis
17. F/u visit 1 bloodwork
18. F/u visit 1 urinalysis
19. F/u visit 2 bloodwork
20. F/u visit 2 urinalysis

21. F/u visit 3 bloodwork

22. F/u visit 3 urinalysis

23. F/u visit 4 bloodwork

24. F/u visit 4 urinalysis

25. F/u visit 5 bloodwork

26. F/u visit 5 urinalysis

27. F/u visit 6 bloodwork

28. F/u visit 6 urinalysis

SECTION 3: QUESTIONNAIRE

29. Prior to starting the SKD diet, did you have any previous diet restrictions? Did you follow a specific diet or eating style such as vegetarian, vegan, etc? (open text box).

30. Rate your level of compliance with the SKD diet. (Response options: (1) 0-25% compliant (follow less than 1 meal a day on average), (2) 26-50% compliant (up to half of daily meals follow the diet), (3) 51-75% compliant (most meals daily follow the diet) and (4) 76-100% compliant (most to all meals and snacks follow the diet daily).

31. Rate your level of compliance with Albutrix. (Response options: (1) 0-25% compliant (take Albutrix as directed less than 2 days per week), (2) 26-50% compliant (take Albutrix as directed 3 days per week), (3) 51-75% compliant (take Albutrix as directed 4 days per week) and (4) 76-100% compliant (take Albutrix as directed 5-7 days per week).

32. Rate your level of compliance with Microtrix. (Response options: (1) 0-25% compliant (take Microtrix as directed less than 2 days per week), (2) 26-50% compliant (take Microtrix as directed 3 days per week), (3) 51-75% compliant (take Microtrix as directed 4 days per week) and (4) 76-100% compliant (take Microtrix as directed 5-7 days per week).

33. Rate the taste of the food in the Stopping Kidney Disease diet. (Response options: (1) Poor (2) Fair (3) Good (4) Great)

34. Any comments you'd like to share about the taste of the food in the Stopping Kidney Disease diet? (open-ended response)

35. Rate the food variety in the Stopping Kidney Disease diet. (Response options: (1) Poor (2) Fair (3) Good (4) Great)

36. Any comments you'd like to share about the food variety in the Stopping Kidney Disease diet? (open-ended response)

37. Rate the ease of preparing meals in the Stopping Kidney Disease diet. (Response options: (1) Poor (2) Fair (3) Good (4) Great)

38. Any comments you'd like to share about the ease of preparing meals in the Stopping Kidney Disease diet? (open-ended response)

39. How can we improve the Stopping Kidney Disease diet? (open-ended response)

40. What is one thing we can do with the Stopping Kidney Disease diet that would help you be more compliant with the diet (following the diet for more meals and snacks each day? (open-ended response)

41. What thoughts/comments would you like to share about Albutrix? (open-ended response)

42. What thoughts/comments would you like to share about Microtrix? (open-ended response)

43. How can we improve Albutrix? (open-ended response)

44. How can we improve Microtrix? (open-ended response)

45. Have you noticed any health-related changes since starting the Stopping Kidney Disease program? If yes, please describe. (yes, no, open-ended comment box)

Appendix D

LAB VALUES COLLECTED

WBC

RBC

RDW

HCT

HGB

MCV

MCH

MCHC

Platelet

Neutrophils

Lymphocytes

Monocytes

Eosinophils

Basophils

Glucose

BUN

Creatinine

BUN/Creatinine Ratio

eGFR

Sodium

Potassium

Chloride

Carbon Dioxide

Calcium

Protein

Albumin

Globulin

Albumin/Globulin Ratio

Bilirubin

ALP

AST

ALT

A1C

Appendix E

Kidneyhood.org dietary program, Albutrix and Microtrix descriptions

The dietary approach used in this pilot study included 3 integrated components:

1. A very low protein diet optimized for kidney disease patients

2. Albutrix S3, S4, or S5

3. Microtrix low serving multivitamin

Descriptions of each component and the dietary strategy used is described.

Kidneyhood.org dietary program

Currently published as the Stopping Kidney Disease Food Guide.

The Kidneyhood.org dietary program is a very low protein diet consisting of the following:

Dietary protein intake of 0.4 grams per kg of ideal body weight while increasing or limiting intake of the following:

Sodium

Plant based phosphorus

Potassium

Advanced glycation end products (AGE's)

Renal acid load

Supplemental calcium

Saturated fats

Supplemental magnesium

Antioxidants

Polyphenols

Dietary nitrates

Fiber

High/Low glycemic index foods

The dietary approach does not require patients to calculate daily dietary values. Patients are compliant when they follow the program. Approximately 80% of patients can follow the program at home without assistance and still achieve measurable results.

Albutrix S3, S4 and S5

Albutrix low nitrogen protein food is a keto acid analog/amino acid medical food used to supplement protein intake and reduce supplemental nitrogen intake. The dietary strategy used is to only supplement what is missing in dietary amino acid intake. First, dietary intake of essential amino acids is calculated for the Kidneyhood. org dietary program. Second, only shortfalls in dietary intake are supplemented. The total from dietary intake and supplemental intake normally meets or exceeds the RDA for each of the 9 essential amino acids.

The valuable benefit of this strategy is the lowest possible waste workloads for diseased kidneys while ensuring RDAs for each essential amino acid are met.

Albutrix is formulated into 3 versions to optimize long term outcomes and reflect the patient's current needs. The Albutrix series is interchangeable so that patients can switch versions based on current blood test results. This strategy allows patients to control intake of supplemental calcium and magnesium.

Albutrix S3 or stage 3 is the first magnesium based keto acid analog. Long-term use of supplemental calcium is no longer recommended for kidney patients (2016 KDOQI) due to risks of accelerated heart disease. Albutrix S3 allows long term use without the risk of supplemental calcium use.

Albutrix S4 or stage 4 is a magnesium/calcium blend consisting of 180 mg of calcium and 180 mg of magnesium for the maximum daily serving. Albutrix S4 allows patients to reduce both calcium and magnesium intake to very low levels.

Albutrix S5 is a 100% calcium-based keto acid analog designed for patients with a GFR below 15. In some late-stage patients, magnesium levels will start to rise. Albutrix S5 allows patients to have a magnesium-free version if needed.

The 3 options allow patients and clinicians to adjust intake as needed to ensure blood test results within normal ranges are achieved and maintained.

Microtrix low serving multivitamin

A similar strategy is used for Microtrix; only shortfalls in dietary intake are supplemented. If dietary intake is 100% of the RDA, then no supplementation is justified. The total intake from the Kidneyhood.org dietary program and Microtrix combine to meet the RDAs.

Higher risk or very patient-specific vitamins or minerals are not supplemented in Microtrix. Vitamin D and iron are not included due the risk of excess intake and wide variation in patient requirements.

Kidneyhood.org Pilot Study References

1. Collaboration GBDCKD. Global, regional, and national burden of chronic kidney disease, 1990-2017: A systematic analysis for the Global Burden of Disease Study 2017. *Lancet.* 2020;395(10225):709-733. DOI: 10.1016/S0140-6736(20)30045-3.

2. Garofalo C, Borrelli S, Liberti ME, et al. Secular trend in GFR decline in non-dialysis CKD based on observational data from standard of care arms of trials. *Am J Kidney Dis.* 2024;83(4):435-444.el. DOI: 10.1053/j.ajkd.2023.09.014.

3. Levene PA, Kristeller L, Manson D. On the character of protein metabolism in chronic nephritis. *J Exp Med.* 1909;11(6):825-38. DOI: 10.1084/jem.11.6.825.

4. Klahr S, Levey AS, Beck GJ, et al. The effects of dietary protein restriction and blood-pressure control on the progression of chronic renal disease. Modification of Diet in Renal Disease Study Group. *N Engl J Med.* 1994;330(13):877-84. DOI: 10.1056/NEJM199403313301301.

5. Rhee CM, Ahmadi SF, Kovesdy CP, Kalantar-Zadeh K. Low-protein diet for conservative management of chronic kidney disease: A systematic review and meta-analysis of controlled trials. *J Cachexia Sarcopenia Muscle.* 2017;9(2):235-245. DOI: 10.1002/jcsm.12264.

6. D'Apolito M, Du X, Pisanelli D, et al. Urea-induced ROS cause endothelial dysfunction in chronic renal failure. *Atherosclerosis.* 2015;239(2):393-400. DOI: 10.1016/j.atherosclerosis.2015.01.034.

7. D'Apolito M, Du X, Zong H, et al. Urea-induced ROS generation causes insulin resistance in mice with chronic renal failure. *J Clin Invest.* 2010;120(1):203-213. DOI: 10.1172/jci37672.

8. Eardley KS, Zehnder D, Quinkler M, et al. The relationship between albuminuria, MCP-1/CCL2, and interstitial macrophages in chronic kidney disease. *Kidney Int.* 2006;69(7):1189-1197. DOI: 10.1038/sj.ki.5000212.

9. Gansevoort RT, de Zeeuw D, de Jong PE. Additive antiproteinuric effect of ACE inhibition and a low-protein diet in human renal disease. *Nephrol Dial Transplant.* 1995;10(4):497-504. DOI: 10.1093/ndt/10.4.497.

10. Walker JD, Bending JJ, Dodds RA, et al. Restriction of dietary protein and progression of renal failure in diabetic nephropathy. *Lancet.* 1989;2(8677):1411-5. DOI: 10.1016/s0140-6736(89)92032-1.

11. Amir S, Kim H, Hu EA, et al. Adherence to plant-based diets and risk of CKD progression and all-cause mortality: Findings from the chronic renal insufficiency cohort (CRIC) study. *Am J Kidney Dis.* 2024;83(5):624-635. DOI: 10.1053/j.ajkd.2023.09.020.

12. Mitch WE. Dietary protein restriction in chronic renal failure: Nutritional efficacy, compliance, and progression of renal insufficiency. *J Am Soc Nephrol.* 1991;2(4):823-31. DOI: 10.1681/ASN.V24823.

13. Chewcharat A, Takkavatakarn K, Wongrattanagorn S, et al. The effects of restricted protein diet supplemented with ketoanalogue on renal function, blood pressure, nutritional status, and chronic kidney disease-mineral and bone disorder in chronic kidney disease patients: A systematic review and meta-analysis. *J Ren Nutr.* 2020;30(3):189-199. DOI: 10.1053/j.jrn.2019.07.005.

14. Li A, Lee H-Y, Lin Y-C. The effect of ketoanalogues on chronic kidney disease deterioration: A meta-analysis. *Nutrients.* 2019;11(5). DOI: 10.3390/nu11050957.

15. Masud T, Young VR, Chapman T, Maroni BJ. Adaptive responses to very low protein diets: The first comparison of ketoacids to essential amino acids. *Kidney Int.* 1994;45(4):1182-1192. DOI: 10.1038/ki.1994.157.

16. Giovannetti S. Answers to ten questions on the dietary treatment of chronic renal failure. *Lancet.* 1986;328(8516):1140-1142. DOI: 10.1016/s0140-6736(86)90542-8.

17. Wrone EM, Carnethon MR, Palaniappan L, Fortmann SP. Association of dietary protein intake and microalbuminuria in healthy adults: Third National Health and Nutrition Examination Survey. *Am J Kid Dis.* 2003;41(3):580-587. DOI: 10.1053/ajkd.2003.50119.

18. Oldrizzi L, Rugiu C, Valvo E, et al. Progression of renal failure in patients with renal disease of diverse etiology on protein-restricted diet. *Kid Int.* 1985;27(3):553-557. DOI: 10.1038/ki.1985.46.

INDEX

Note: **Bold** pages refer tables in the text.

Made in the USA
Las Vegas, NV
25 November 2024

12590979R00096